Essential Bioinformatics and Data Mining

Essential Bioinformatics and Data Mining

Biswajit Brahma
Ph.D. Animal Biotechnology
Assistant Professor
Sher-e-Kashmir University of Agricultural Sciences &
Technology of Jammu, India

Dhirendra Kumar
Ph.D. Animal Genetics & Breeding
Assistant Professor
Sher-e-Kashmir University of Agricultural Sciences &
Technology of Jammu, India

SSPH

SATISH SERIAL PUBLISHING HOUSE
403, Express Tower, Commercial Complex
Azadpur, Delhi-110033 (India)
Phone : 011-27672852, Fax : 91-11-27672046
e-mail : info@satishserial.com, hkjain1975@yahoo.com
Website : www.satishserial.com

Published by :

SATISH SERIAL PUBLISHING HOUSE
403, Express Tower, Commercial Complex, Azadpur, Delhi-110033 (INDIA)
Phone : 011-27672852 Fax : 91-11-27672046
E-mail : info@satishserial.com, hkjain1975@yahoo.com

ISBN 978-93-86200-45-7

Composed, Designed & Printed in India

Preface

With rapid developments of big data challenges in the era of "omics" sciences, bioinformatics is becoming growingly popular and an indispensable component for large amount of sequence information being reported every day at whole genome and transcriptome level. Analysing large biological data sets requires making sense of the data by inferring structure or generalizations from the data. Data mining, the extraction of hidden predictive information from large databases, is becoming an important tool to transform this data into information. In these fields, there is a much-needed development of computational tools to deal with a monumental amount of genomic and post-genomic data, aiming at systems-level understanding in biology. The parallel conference workshop on "Essential Bioinformatics and Data Mining" along the International conference on "Recent trends in bioinformatics and biotechnology for sustainable development", was organized to provide scientists and researchers in the area of computational systems biology and bioinformatics with a forum to share and exchange their knowledge and experiences. The present publication entitled 'Essential Bioinformatics and Data Mining' comprises of 11 chapters as a compilation of invited lectures, presented in the parallel Conference Workshop of Society for Bioinformatics and Biological Sciences (SBBS) at Faculty of Veterinary Sciences and Animal Husbandry, R.S.Pura, Sher-e-Kashmir University of Agricultural Sciences and Technology of Jammu, J&K, India during October 12-13, 2017. Careful efforts have been made in compilation of this publication and error, if any may kindly be pardoned and brought to the notice for further improvement. We hope this present publication will be useful to students and academicians working in the field Bioinformatics, data mining and other related filed.

Editors

List of Contributors

Akhilesh Upgade
Assistant Professor
Dept. of Microbiology
Shree M & N Virani Science
College, Rajkot
Email: aaupgade@vsc.edu.in

Banti Kumar
Division of Statistics and
Computer Science
Faculty of Basic Sciences
Sher-e-Kashmir University
of Agricultural Sciences &
Technology of Jammu, India

B. Brahma
Assistant Professor
Division of Livestock
Production & Management
Sher-e-Kashmir University
of Agricultural Sciences &
Technology of Jammu, India

Budhayash Gautam
Assistant Professor (Sr. Grade)
Department of Computational
Biology & Bioinformatics
Sam Higginbottom Institute
of Agriculture, Technology &
Sciences (SHUATS)
Allahabad, Uttar Pradesh

Dhirendra Kumar
Assistant Professor
Divison of Animal Genetics and
Breeding, Sher-e-Kashmir
University of Agricultural Sciences
& Technology of Jammu, India

Dibyendu Chakraborty
Assistant Professor
Divison of Animal Genetics
and Breeding
Sher-e-Kashmir University
of Agricultural Sciences &
Technology of Jammu,
India

Diksha Bhadwal
School of Biotechnology
Sher-e-Kashmir University
of Agricultural Sciences &
Technology of Jammu,
India

Gyanendra Kumar Rai
Assistant Professor
School of Biotechnology
Sher-e-Kashmir University
of Agricultural Sciences &
Technology of Jammu,
India

Lopamudra Chakraborty
MGDC, SKMU-Dumka

Manish Sharma
Associate Professor (Statistics)
Division of Statistics and
Computer Science
Faculty of Basic Sciences
Sher-e-Kashmir University of
Agricultural Sciences &
Technology of Jammu,
India
Email:manshstat@gmail.com

Nishant Kumar
Assistant Professor
Divison of Animal Genetics
and Breeding
Sher-e-Kashmir University
of Agricultural Sciences &
Technology of Jammu,
India

Nusrat Nabi Khan
Divison of Animal Genetics
and Breeding
SK Universitiy of Agricultural
Science and Technology
Srinagar, India

P. Kumarasamy
Professor and Head,
Bioinformatics Centre & ARIS
Cell, Madras Veterinary College,
Chennai-600 007 India,
Email: pksamy2000@gmail.com

Rakhshan Jeelani
Division of Livestock
Production & Management
Sher-e-Kashmir University
of Agricultural Sciences &
Technology of Jammu, India

Raman Kumar Taggar
Professor & Head, Divison of
Animal Genetics and Breeding,
Sher-e-Kashmir University of
Agricultural Sciences &
Technology of Jammu,
India

Sachinandan De
Animal Genomics Laboratory,
Animal Biotechnology Centre,
National Dairy Research Institute,
Karnal, Haryana, India

Satendra Singh
Assistant Professor
Department of Computational
Biology & Bioinformatics
JIBB, Sam Higginbottom
University of Agriculture,
Technology and Sciences
Allahabad, India

Simran Singh
Division of Animal Genetics
and Breeding, Sher-e-Kashmir
University of Agricultural Sciences
& Technology of Jammu, India

Sreshti Bagati
School of Biotechnology
Sher-e-Kashmir University
of Agricultural Sciences &
Technology of Jammu, India

Mrs. Vibha Raj Shanti
School of Biotechnology
Sher-e-Kashmir University
of Agricultural Sciences &
Technology of Jammu, India

Vikas Mahajan
Assistant Professor
ILFC, Sher-e-Kashmir University
of Agricultural Sciences &
Technology of Jammu, India

❑❑❑

Contents

Chapter 1

Application of Bioinformatics for Agriculture and Animal Science

P. Kumarasamy

Essential Bioinformatics is a concise word given specifically for life science students; the basics of bioinformatics are of the state-of-the-art computational tools available to solve biological research problems. Key areas of bioinformatics are biological databases, sequence alignment, gene and promoter prediction, molecular phylogenetics, structural bioinformatics, genomics, and proteomics.

With a large number of prokaryotic and eukaryotic genomes completely sequenced and more forthcoming, access to the genomic information and synthesizing it for the discovery of new knowledge have become central themes of modern biological research. Mining the genomic information requires the use of sophisticated computational tools. It therefore becomes imperative for the new generation of biologists to be familiar with many bioinformatics programs and databases to tackle the new challenges in the genomic era. To meet this goal, institutions in the United States and around the world are now offering graduate and undergraduate students bioinformatics-related courses to introduce them to relevant computational tools necessary for the genomic research. Therefore, many biological terms, such as nucleic acids, amino acids, genes, transcription, and translation, are used without further explanation. This lead paper will cover the areas like Biological databases, sequence alignment, genes and promoter prediction, molecular phylogenetics, structural bioinformatics, and genomics and proteomics use of data mining.

Biological databases contain a wide variety of data. Consider storing in a database the operational details of a single cell organism. At minimum one would need to encode the following.

- Genome: DNA sequence and gene locations
- Proteome: the organism's full complement of proteins, not necessarily a direct mapping from its genes
- Metabolic pathways: linked biochemical reactions involving multiple proteins, small molecules and protein- protein interactions
- Regulatory pathways: the mechanism by which the expression of some genes into proteins, such as transcription factors, influences the expression of other genes-includes protein-DNA interactions. In fact, such a database exists for part of what is known of the widely-studied model organism. Recording the diversity of data in the previous paragraph obviously requires a rich relational schema with multiple, interacting relational tables. At present we do not have complete knowledge of the workings of any organism, biological databases often encode a variety of types of laboratory data that provide further insight into organism behavior. This may include data from the following high throughput techniques:
    - Gene expression microarrays: measure the degree to which each gene is being transcribed into messenger RNA (mRNA) under various conditions
    - Proteomics (primarily mass spectrometry): provides insight into which proteins are present in significant concentrations, as well as protein-protein interactions
    - Metabolomics: measures the concentrations of small molecules (i.e., those with low molecular weight) in a sample
    - Single-nucleotide polymorphism (SNP) measurements: SNP patterns are used as a surrogate for complete DNA sequences of multiple individuals, e.g. human patients - SNPs are single-base positions in DNA where individuals commonly differ
    - DNA chip technology for Genome Wide Association studies.

Data mining

Data mining, *the extraction of hidden predictive information from large databases,* is a powerful new technology with great potential to help companies focus on the most important information in their data warehouses. Data mining tools predict future trends and behaviors, allowing businesses to make proactive, knowledge-driven decisions. The automated, prospective analyses offered by data mining move beyond the analyses of past events provided by retrospective tools typical of decision support systems. Data mining tools can answer business questions that traditionally were too time consuming to resolve. They scour databases for hidden patterns, finding predictive information that experts may miss because it lies outside their expectations.

Data mining is ready for application in the business community because it is supported by three technologies that are now sufficiently mature:

- Massive data collection
- Powerful multiprocessor computers
- Data mining algorithms

The Scope of Data Mining

Data mining techniques can yield the benefits of automation on existing software and hardware platforms, and can be implemented on new systems as existing platforms are upgraded and new products developed. The most commonly used techniques in data mining are:

- **Artificial neural networks**: Non-linear predictive models that learn through training and resemble biological neural networks in structure.
- **Decision trees**: Tree-shaped structures that represent sets of decisions. These decisions generate rules for the classification of a dataset. Specific decision tree methods include Classification and Regression Trees (CART) and Chi Square Automatic Interaction Detection (CHAID).
- **Genetic algorithms**: Optimization techniques that use process such as genetic combination, mutation, and natural selection in a design based on the concepts of evolution.
- **Nearest neighbor method**: A technique that classifies each record in a dataset based on a combination of the classes of the k record(s) most similar to it in a historical dataset (where $k \geq 1$). Sometimes called the k-nearest neighbor technique.

- **Rule induction**: The extraction of useful if-then rules from data based on statistical significance.

GENOME SELECTION

Genomic selection offers many advantages with regard to improving the rate of genetic gain in dairy cattle breeding programs. The most important factors that contribute to faster genetic gain include, A greater accuracy of predicted genetic merit for young animals. A shorter generation interval because of heavier use of young, genetically superior males and females. An increased intensity of selection because breeders can use genomic testing to screen a larger group of potentially elite animals. By increasing the accuracy and intensity of selection and shortening the generation interval, the rate of genetic progress for economically important dairy traits can be approximately doubled.

In practice, genomic selection refers to selection decisions based on genomic estimated breeding values (GEBV). These GEBV are calculated by estimating SNP effects from prediction equations, which are derived from a subset of animals in the population (i.e., a reference population) that have SNP genotypes and phenotypes for traits of interest.

Genomic selection has been rapidly adopted by the dairy cattle breeding industry, particularly in the Holstein breed, and its use in other cattle breeds and livestock species is under investigation. In this transition period, strategies to implement genomic selection have been rather prudent, although the largest gains could be obtained by extensive use of genomic information. Success of this new selection method critically dependson the availability of large databases of phenotypes and genotypes. Genomic selection also appears to be a promising tool to curb inbreeding rates because it allows exploitation of within-family genetic variance from the earliest selection stages. However, to be effective, breeders must consider using a diversied panel of genomically evaluated bulls, both to mitigate the risk of using bulls with poor merit and to limit the erosion of genetic diversity. To this end, the further development and application of tools, such as genomic optimal contribution selection, are critical for sustainable use of genetic resources. Estimating the genetic potential of selection candidates, the rate of genetic gain can be increased from 15 per cent to 60 per cent, depending on the trait chosen.

DESIGNER LIVESTOCK AND CROP

We can design the animals and plants using gene editing CRISPR/ Cas9 system to target a gene called POLLED in the cells of dairy cattle, changing it to a version that resembles that of the hornless beef cattle, targeting the gene for myostatin, a negative regulator of muscle growth, to increase the muscle mass of cattle and pigs, GM chickens that express an RNA decoy that distracts the avian influenza virus from replication, the transfection of viral genetic fragments into an animal's genome to trigger the inhibitory phenomenon known as RNA interference (RNAi) for disease resistance. Increasing twining in sheep, increasing the milk yield, expression of therapeutic agents in milk etc., would be novel ideas put into use for benefit of human.

CONCLUSION

Multi-relational data mining tools have been applied to a variety of biological tasks. Nevertheless, the breadth of inter-related data types in the introduction is significantly greater than in any of the specific applications. Furthermore, with the growth in systems biology, the breadth and relational structure of biological databases will only increase. Therefore, biological databases provide a major challenge for multi-relational data mining. Already, data mining researchers should be more ambitious in applying multi-relational algorithms to larger and more diverse databases. For example, we should be integrating data on DNA (SNPs), mRNA (from gene expression microarrays), proteins (from mass spectrometry) and metabolomics into multi-relational analyses. We should be drawing on relevant text sources as well. Stretching ourselves in this manner in applications is sure to reveal new research directions in the development of multi-relational data mining algorithms for the benefit of human society.

Hence, the knowledge of Genomic and Bioinformatics tools are very important for the Scientist in Agriculture and Animal Science. By using these tools, the improvement of productivity and conservation of Indigenous varieties will be possible in future.

❑❑❑

Chapter 2

Bioinformatics Resources for Analysis of Genomics and Proteomics Data

Satendra Singh

The goal of agriculture and animal genomics is to understand the genetic and molecular basis of all biological processes in plants and animal that are relevant to the specie. This understanding is fundamental to allow efficient exploitation of biological resources in the development of new cultivars with improved quality and reduced economic and environmental costs. This knowledge is also vital for the development of new verities. Traits considered of primary interest are, pathogen and abiotic stress resistance, quality traits , and reproductive traits determining yield. Current genome programs generate a large amount of data that will require processing, storage and distribution to the multinational research community. The data include not only sequence information, but information on mutations, markers, maps, functional discoveries, etc. In this chapter, we provide an informatics how different approaches, tools and databases can be utilized for the animal breeding and genetics.

Bioinformatics is applied for

- Crop improvement
- Insect resistance
- Improve nutritional quality
- Development of Drought resistance varieties
- Vetinary Science
- Microbial genome applications

The field of bioinformatics emerged as a tool to facilitate biological discoveries more than 20 years ago. With the development of Human Genome Project (HGP), the data of biology increased fabulously and marvelously. The ability to capture, manage, process, analyze and interpret data became more important than ever. Bioinformatics and computers can help scientists to solve it.

Bioinformatics which is coming with HGP brings together the fields of life science, computer science and statistics and strives to understand medical and biological systems by the creative application of statistics and computer analysis. Bioinformatics is the use of computer technology to help scientists keep track of the genetic information they find. Using computers, researchers can gather, store, analyze and compare biological data with great speed and accuracy.

Imagine studying gene structures without the help of a computer. It would take many years to compare the 15,000 genes of Arabidopsis to the genes of a similar plant. And keeping track of the 100,000 genes of a human being would be inconceivable. With computers, the process of comparison is automated. By storing information as it is discovered, computers ease the immense job of genome mapping. But computers can analyze as well as store information. They can be used to construct models that reduce the need for experimentation. In this way, biotechnology has become more efficient. Scientists are able to use fairly reliable computer-assisted predictions of test results on genetic modifications. This complements the time-consuming process involved in growing out every modified plant in the laboratory or greenhouse to test for the desired modification.

BIOINFORMATICS IN AGRICULTURE

Bioinformatics today has entered every major discipline in biology. In genomics, Bioinformatics has aided in genome sequencing, and has shown its success in locating the genes, in phylogenetic comparison and in the detection of transcription factor binding sites of the genes (Liu et al.,1995; This G et al.,2002), just to name a few. Microarray technology has opened the world of transcriptomics in front 'biologists (Spellman et al., 1998; Eisen et al., 1998). Bioinformatics provides analytical tools for microarray data. These tools range from image the processing techniques that read out the data, to the visualization tools that provide a first-sight hint to the biologists; from preprocessing techniques (Durbin et al., 2002) that remove the systematic noise in the data to the clustering methods (Eisen et al., 1998; Sheng et al., 2003) that reveal genes that behave similarly under different experimental conditions. In proteomics, bioinformatics helps in the study of protein structures and the discovery of sequence sites where protein-protein interactions take place. To help understanding biology at the system level, bioinformatics begins to show promise in unravelling genetic networks (Segal et al., 2003). Finally, in the study of metabolome, bioinformatics is used to study the dynamics in a cell, and thus to simulate the cellular interactions.

Plant life plays important and diverse roles in our society, our economy, and our global environment. Especially crop is the most important plants to us. Feeding the increasing world population is a challenge for modern plant biotechnology. Crop yields have increased during the last century and will continue to improve as agronomy re-assorting the enhanced breeding and develop new biotechnological-engineered strategies. The onset of genomics is providing massive information to improve crop phenotypes. The accumulation of sequence data allows detailed genome analysis by usingfriendly database access and information retrieval. Genetic and molecular genome co linearity allows efficient transfer of data revealing extensive conservation of genome organization between species. The goals of genome research are the identification of the sequenced genes and the deduction of their functions by metabolic analysis and reverses genetic screens of gene knockouts. Over 20% of the predicted genes occur as cluster of related genes generating a considerable proportion of gene families. Multiple alignment provides a method to estimate the number of genes in gene families allowing the identification of previously undescribed genes. This information enables new strategies to study gene expression patterns in plants. Available in formation from news technologies, as the database stored DNA microarray expression data, will help plant biology functional genomics. Expressed sequence tags (ESTs) also give the opportunity to perform "digital northern" comparison of gene expression levels providing initial clues toward unknown regulatory phenomena. Crop plant networks collections of databases and bioinformatics resources for crop plants genomics have been

Sequence analysis

Sequence analysis can be used to assign function to genes and proteins by the study of the similarities between the compared sequences, revealing the evolution and genetic diversity of organisms and Function annotation of genes.

Software Name	Description
ALIGN	This tool is used to compare 2 sequences, have options for both global and local alignment
CENSOR	CENSOR is a software tool which screens query sequences against a reference collection of repeats and "censors" (masks) homologous portions with masking symbols, as well
CLUSTALW2	General purpose multiple sequence alignment program for DNA or proteins. It produces biologically meaningful multiple sequence alignments of divergent sequences. It calculates the best match for the selected sequences, and lines them up so that the identities, similarities and differences can be seen. Evolutionary relationships can be seen via viewing Cladograms or Phylograms.
Genewise	Aligns two sequences under the assumption that the sequences share a number of colinear blocks of conservation separated by potentially large and varied lengths of DNA in the two sequences.
Kalign	A fast and accurate multiple sequence alignment algorithm.
PromoterWise	The Wise2 form compares a protein sequence to a genomic DNA sequence, allowing for introns and frameshifting errors.
SAPS	SAPS evaluates by statistical criteria a wide variety of protein sequence properties. Properties considered include compositional biases, clusters and runs of charge and other amino acid types, different kinds and extents of repetitive structures, locally periodic motifs, and anomalous spacings between identical residue types.
T-coffee	T-Coffee is a multiple sequence alignment program. It allows to combine results obtained with several alignment methods.

Transeq	Transeq translates nucleic acid sequences to the corresponding peptide sequence. It can translate in any of the 3 forward or three reverse sense frames, or in all three forward or reverse frames, or in all six frames.
COBALT	COBALT is a multiple sequence alignment tool that finds a collection of pairwise constraints derived from conserved domain database, protein motif database, and sequence similarity, using RPS-BLAST, BLASTP, and PHI-BLAST.
Genome Workbench	NCBI Genome Workbench is an integrated application for viewing and analyzing sequence data. With Genome Workbench, you can view data in publically available sequence databases at NCBI, and mix this data with your own private data.
ORF Finder	The ORF Finder (Open Reading Frame Finder) is a graphical analysis tool which finds all open reading frames of a selectable minimum size in a user's sequence or in a sequence already in the database.
Primer - BLAST	To help users make primers that are specific to the input PCR template. It uses Primer3 to design PCR primers and then submits them to BLAST search against user-selected database.
VecScreen	VecScreen is a system for quickly identifying segments of a nucleic acid sequence that may be of vector origin.
WU-BLAST	WU-BLAST2 stands for Washington University Basic Local Alignment Search Tool Version 2.0. The emphasis of this tool is to find regions of sequence similarity quickly, with minimum loss of sensitivity.
SeWeR	SEquence analysis using WEb Resources, is an integrated portal to common web-based services in bioinformatics.
Motif Search	Making the search for promoters and inverted repeats.
DNA Translator	Sequence translation from DNA to Proteins.
Non coding RNA Gene Finder	Search for Non coding RNA Genes.
TransTerm	TransTerm searches for Á-independent terminators in the vicinity of annotated genes.

QRNA	QRNA determined from the nature of the substitutions in blastn alignments, whether it could be in homologous sequences is a non- coding RNA (ncRNA).
Clustalformatter 5	Sequence Analysis
BioEdit	BioEdit is a biological sequence alignment editor written for Windows 95/98/NT/2000/XP. An intuitive multiple document interface with convenient features makes alignment and manipulation of sequences relatively easy on your desktop computer.
FASTA	FASTA (pronounced FAST-AYE) stands for FAST-ALL, reflecting the fact that it can be used for a fast protein comparison or a fast nucleotide comparison. This program achieves a high level of sensitivity for similarity searching at high speed.
HMMER	HMMER is used for searching sequence databases for homologs of protein sequences, and for making protein sequence alignments. It implements methods using probabilistic models called "profile hidden Markov models".
JAligner	An open source Java implementation of the Smith-Waterman algorithm with Gotoh's improvement for biological local pairwise sequence alignment using the affine gap penalty model.
JSTRING	Java Search for Tandem Repeats IN Genomes, is graphical and interactive implementation of the algorithm STRING.
NCBI BLAST	The Basic Local Alignment Search Tool (BLAST) finds regions of local similarity between sequences. The program compares nucleotide or protein sequences to sequence databases and calculates the statistical significance of matches.
Gene Runner/ Motif Runner	Motif based Sequence Analysis
GoCore	GoCore is a free bioinformatics tool for protein sequence alignment and analysis. It operates as an Excel add-in, creating additional menu items that perform the bioinformatics analyses and uses Excel's convenient user interface to provide useful visualizations.

MAFFT	Multiple Alignment
MAUVE	Mauve is a system for efficiently constructing multiple genome alignments in the presence of large-scale evolutionary events such as rearrangement and inversion.
MEME Suite	MEME is a tool for discovering motifs in a group of related DNA or protein sequences.
CORAL (CDTree)	Aligning Core Conserved Regions, a powerful tool to aid in the classification of protein sequences and investigate their evolutionary relationships.
BlastAlign	BlastAlign: a program that uses blast to align nucleotide sequences that have large indels (INsertions/DELetions) or are otherwise difficult to align.
ARB software	The ARB software is a graphically oriented package comprising various tools for sequence database handling and data analysis.
ACUA	ACUA is a Visual Basic based interface for the Insilico codon analysis. This tool provides various unique features like, Nucleotide analysis, statistical codon analysis, Positional nucleotide analysis and interactive analysis of result.
AnnHyb	AnnHyb is a tool for working with and managing nucleotide sequences in multiple formats. The features include sequence viewer, sequence editor, sequence annotation, format conversion, oligonucleotides alignment, restriction analysis, pattern searching, retrieval from servers, multi-alignment viewer, consensus determination.
SOAP2	SOAP has been in evolution from a single alignment tool to a tool package that provides full solution to next generation sequencing data analysis.
ACT (Artemis Comparison Tool)	ACT is a DNA sequence comparison viewer written in Java. It is based on the software for Artemis, the genome viewer and annotation tool.

Phylogenetic analysis

Phylogenetic analysis is the process to determine the evolutionary relationships between organisms. Phylogenetic trees determining evolutionary relationships includes matching patterns in nucleic acid and protein sequences.

Software Name	Description
PHYLIP	PHYLIP is a free package of programs for inferring phylogenies. It is distributed as source code, documentation files, and a number of different types of executables.
PAML	PAML is a package of programs for phylogenetic analyses of DNA or protein sequences using maximum likelihood. It is maintained and distributed for academic use free of charge by Ziheng Yang.
Batwing	Phylogenetic Analysis (UNIX/LINUX Software)
Bayes Phylogenies	The program allows a range of models of gene sequence evolution, models for morphological traits, models for rooted trees, gamma and beta distributed rate-heterogeneity, and implements a 'mixture model' (Pagel and Meade, 2004) that allows the user to fit more than one model of sequence evolution, without partitioning the data.
Bayes Traits	The program allows a range of models of gene sequence evolution, models for morphological traits, models for rooted trees, gamma and beta distributed rate-heterogeneity, and implements a 'mixture model' (Pagel and Meade, 2004) that allows the user to fit more than one model of sequence evolution, without partitioning the data.
BEAST	BEAST is a cross-platform program for Bayesian MCMC analysis of molecular sequences. It is entirely orientated towards rooted, time-measured phylogenies inferred using strict or relaxed molecular clock models.
Bosque	Gblocks is a tool for the selection of conserved blocks from multiple alignments for their use in phylogenetic analysis. It eliminates poorly aligned positions and divergent regions of an alignment of DNA or protein sequences.

ClustalW	ClustalW is a general purpose multiple sequence alignment program for DNA or proteins. It produces biologically meaningful multiple sequence alignments of divergent sequences.

Annotation

Annotation software system design to find the genes (places in the DNA sequence that encode a protein), the transfer RNA, and other features, and to make initial assignments of function to those genes.

Software Name	Description
Synteny	Synteny compares two genomes with each other using the famous mummer software package. The DNA sequences are first compared at the DNA level using Nucmer
Artemis	DNA Sequence Viewer and Annotation Tool that allows visualisation of sequence features and the results of analyses within the context of the sequence, and also its six-frame translation.
Protein Finder	Protein finder is a gendetector. The program finds genes by performing blastx searches of the input sequence against non redundant database.
Glimmer	Glimmer is a system for finding genes in microbial DNA, especially the genomes of bacteria, archaea, and viruses.
GlimmerHMM	GlimmerHMM is a new gene finder based on a Generalized Hidden Markov Model (GHMM). It also utilizes Interpolated Markov Models for the coding and noncoding models . Currently, GlimmerHMM's GHMM structure includes introns of each phase, intergenic regions, and four types of exons (initial, internal, final, and single).
tRNAscan	The program identifies 99-100% of transfer RNA genes in DNA sequence while giving less than one false positive per 15 gigabases.
Boxer	Boxer searches for Box Elements in genomic DNA. Box elements are a certain type of repeat region that only occurs in few species.
FingerPRINTScan	FingerPRINTScan is a tool that classifies sequences using the family definitions that are present in the

	PRINTS database. It is particularly good at detecting distant evolutionary relationships.
Inquisitor	The Inquisitor examines input protein sequence and identify whether or not it corresponds to a sequence in Integr8 (complete proteomes only) and the UniProt Knowledgebase.
InterProScan	The InterPro database integrates PROSITE, PRINTS, Pfam, ProDom, SMART, TIGRFAMs, PIR superfamily, SUPERFAMILY Gene3D, PANTHER and HAMAP databases. InterPro data is distributed in XML format and it is freely available under the InterPro Consortium copyright.
Phobius	This server is for prediction of transmembrane topology and signal peptides from the amino acid sequence of a protein.
PPSearch	This server searches query sequence for protein motifs, rapidly compare query protein sequence against all patterns. stored in the PROSITE pattern database and determine what the function of an uncharacterised protein is.
Pratt	This tool allows the user to search for patterns conserved in sets of unaligned protein sequences.
Radar	RADAR stands for Rapid Automatic Detection and Alignment of Repeats in protein sequences. Radar is used as an automatic algorithm, for segmenting your query sequence into repeats, it identifies short composition biased as well as gapped approximate repeats and complex repeat architectures involving many different types of repeats in your query sequence.
Proteax	Proteax software suite is used to handle modified proteins and protein derivatives.

Structural analysis

Structural analysis used for determination of a protein's 2D/3D structure is crucial in the study of its function.

Software Name	Description
RasMol	RasMol is a computer program written for molecular graphics visualization intended and used primarily for the depiction and exploration of biological macromolecule structures, such as those found in the Protein Data Bank.
QuteMol	QuteMol is an open source, interactive, molecular visualization system used for studying 3D shape and structure of large molecules or complex proteins
PyMol	PyMOL is a powerful and comprehensive molecular visualization product for rendering and animating 3D molecular structures.
MeshLab	MeshLab is an open source, portable, and extensible system for the processing and editing of unstructured 3D triangular meshes.
Chimera	UCSF Chimera is a highly extensible program for interactive visualization and analysis of molecular structures and related data, including density maps, supramolecular assemblies, sequence alignments, docking results, trajectories, and conformational ensembles.
SwissPDB Viewer	Swiss-PdbViewer is an application that provides a user friendly interface allowing to analyze several proteins at the same time. The proteins can be superimposed in order to deduce structural alignments and compare their active sites or any other relevant parts. Amino acid mutations, H-bonds, angles and distances between atoms are easy to obtain thanks to the intuitive graphic and menu interface
Molekel	Molekel is a free and open-source multiplatform molecular visualization program
Cytospace	Cytoscape is an open source bioinformatics software platform for visualizing molecular interaction networks and integrating these interactions with gene expression profiles and other state data.

BioClipse	Molecular Editor
Avogadro	Avogadro is a 3D molecular structure editor used for editing three-dimensional molecular compositions indicating molecule from every conceivable angle and perspective.
Jmol	Jmol is an open-source Java viewer for three-dimensional chemical structures, with features for chemicals, crystals, materials and biomolecules.
Ascalaph Designer	Ascalaph Designer provides the methods to build and edit molecular models, geometry optimization, molecular dynamics simulations.
GROMACS	GROMACS (GROningenMAchine for Chemical Simulations) is a molecular dynamics simulation package designed for biomolecular systems such as proteins and lipids.
MDynaMix	MDynaMix (Molecular Dynamics of Mixtures) is a general purpose molecular dynamics software package for simulations mixtures of molecules, interacting by AMBER/CHARMM like force fields in a periodic boundary conditions.
TINKER	The TINKER molecular modeling software is a complete and general package for molecular mechanics and dynamics, with some special features for biopolymers.
NAMD	NAMD is a parallel molecular dynamics code designed for high-performance simulation of large biomolecular systems.
DaliLite	DaliLite is a program for pairwise structure comparison and for structure database searching. It is a standalone version of the search engine of the popular Dali server.
EMSearch	Emsearch is a search tool for electron microscopy depositions.
MaxSprout	MaxSprout is a fast database algorithm for generating protein backbone and side chain co-ordinates from a C(alpha) trace.
MSDfold	MSD Fold is a secondary structure matching tool. It also compares protein chains/structures and look for similar ones in the whole PDB archive or among SCOP domains.

MSDpro	MSD pro is a java applet tool that allows you to construct complex relational queries on the PDBe, without needing to know the arrangement of the data within the database, or the language in which such queries are usually written, SQL.
PDBeSite	PDBeSite is a tool which allows the ability to search the active site database based on ligand (eg ATP) or active site (eg CYS CYSCYS CYS) information.
NMR Representatives	NMR Representatives is a search tool for NMR elucidated structures in the PDB.
PDBE Services	PDBE Services is a complete list and summary of all the tools and services the Protein Databank in Europe (PDBe) group have to offer.
PQS	Parallel Quantum Solutions (PQS) provides parallel computers with integrated software for high-performance computational chemistry.
PQS - Quick	PQS-Quick ia a structural analysis tool which quickly retrives protcin quaternary structure information from PDB ID code.
PROCOGNATE	PROCOGNATE is a database of cognate ligands for the domains of enzyme structures in CATH, SCOP and Pfam.
Tempura	Tempura is a function prediction tool and local structural comparison service. It uses the "reverse template" approach published as part of the ProFunc server but has been modified to allow the user to specify the amino acids to be used in the template generation process.
PDBeFOLD	PDBeFold (also known as SSM) is an interactive service for comparing protein structures in 3D. This service provides pairwise and multiple comparison and 3D alignment of protein structures, examination of a protein structure for similarity with the whole PDB archive or SCOP archive.
Receptor Binding Domain Finder	The receptor binding domain finder tries to detect domains in a protein that might be involved in protein-protein interaction by analyzing the amino acid sequence only.

References

JianXue1, Shoujing Zhao, Yanlong Liang, ChunxiHou, Jianhua Wang Bioinformatics and its Applications ion Agriculture.

Durbin, B.P., Hardin, J.S., Hawkins, D.M., Rocke, D.M. (2002). A variance-stabilizing transformation for gene-expression microarray data, Bioinformatics, 18(Suppl. 1): s105.

Eisen, M.B., Spellman, P.T., Brown, P.O., Botstein, D. (1998). Cluster analysis and display of genome-wide expression paterns, ProcNatlAcadSci (USA), 95: 14 863.

Segal, E., Shapira, M., Regev, A., Pe'er, D., Botstein, D., Koller, D., Friedman, N. (2003). Module networks: identifying regulatory modules and their condition-specific regulators from gene expression data. Nat Gen, 34(2):166.

□□□

Chapter 3

Statistical Methods for Data Analysis using SPSS

Manish Sharma and Banti Kumar

INTRODUCTION

Statistics has played a vital role in Veterinary, Agriculture, Medical and allied Sciences starting from planning of the experiment to the analysis of data. The experimentation comprises of two major components viz., designing the experiment (or the way of generating the data) and the analysis of data generated to draw meaningful and valid conclusions. It is through statistical packages only, the drawn results and designs could be developed by graphics, which is simpler to understand even by a layman.

In order to make our research more competitive, the modern statistical methodologies are required for the collection and analysis of data and the interpretation of results. A wide variety of proprietary software packages such as Statistical Analysis System (SAS), Statistical Package for Social Sciences (SPSS), SYSTAT, JMP, GENSTAT, GLIM, MINITAB, S-PLUS, STATISTICA etc. MS-Excels is also very useful to solve a wide type of problems. The free online available software packages are Libre Office cal, PSPP, R and Epilnfo. Here, it is not possible to discuss all in details. So, in this chapter the SPSS software package is discussed which, is a very comprehensive and widely available package for statistical analysis.

SPSS (originally standing for 'Statistical Package for the Social Sciences) but now '(Statistical Product and Service Solutions)' or '(Superior performing Statistical Software)' is one of the leading programmes for managing and analyzing social and scientific data. It was one of the earliest statistical package with version1 being released in 1968, well before the advent of computers. SPSS is now one of the most widely accepted statistical analysis package used worldwide.

SPSS includes the following

- Comprehensive statistical capabilities, including descriptive statistics, simulations and distributions, elementary inferential statistics, analysis of variance, regression, analysis of categorical data, multivariate analysis, non-parametric, control charts and time series analysis.
- A menu-driven interface providing easy access to SPSS statistical, graphical and data management capabilities.
- A data window permitting data entry, editing, and browsing in a spreadsheet like display.
- The ability to import and export data, including data from excel.

Feature of SPSS Software

- One of the most powerful statistical packages that is also easy to use.
- Can use either with menus or syntax files
- It includes a full range of data management system and editing tools
- It provides in-depth statistical capabilities
- More powerful then MINITAB
- SPSS is a powerful and versatile tool that will enhance their learning experience.
- One of the most widely used statistical packages in academia
- It offers complete plotting, reporting and presentation features

There are a number of different types of windows of SPSS the most common in used are as

i) **Data Editor Window** is the first window you encounter while clicking on the icon of the SPSS which, is used to define and enter your data and to perform statistical procedures.

ii) **Output Window** displays the results of the statistical tests.

iii) **Syntax Window** can be used to keep a record of the operations that you perform on your data. This window will be open automatically when someone clicks a **Paste** function of the dialogue box.

These windows can be saved. Basic information on these windows is summarized as.

Windows	File Suffix	Function
Editor	.sav	Used to define, enter, and edit your data and to run statistical tests
Output	.spo	Contains the results of the statistical procedures
Syntax	.sps	This window is activated when you click on the Paste function and records a record of the operations that are "pasted." Although this is beyond the goals of these lessons, you may want to know that SPSS commands can actually be run from this window.

The utility of this statistical software has been discussed with the help of numerical examples in the following sections which include:

a) Descriptive Statistics

b) Normality of the data

c) Correlation

d) Regression Analysis (Simple and Multiple)

e) Tests for one sample and two sample means, paired t test

f) Chi Square for independence of attributes

g) Analysis of Statistical Designs such as

   i) One way ANOVA

   ii) Two way ANOVA

   iii) Three way ANOVA

A. Descriptive Statistics

Example: Following data were obtained from grassland community for number of seeds per plant(X).

X: 29 35 29 19 39 46 59 41 51 29 37 49 63 67

Obtain various types of summary statistics.

SPSS Commands (Step by Step)

Analyze, Descriptive Statistics, X (Put under variables), Option, Continue and OK.

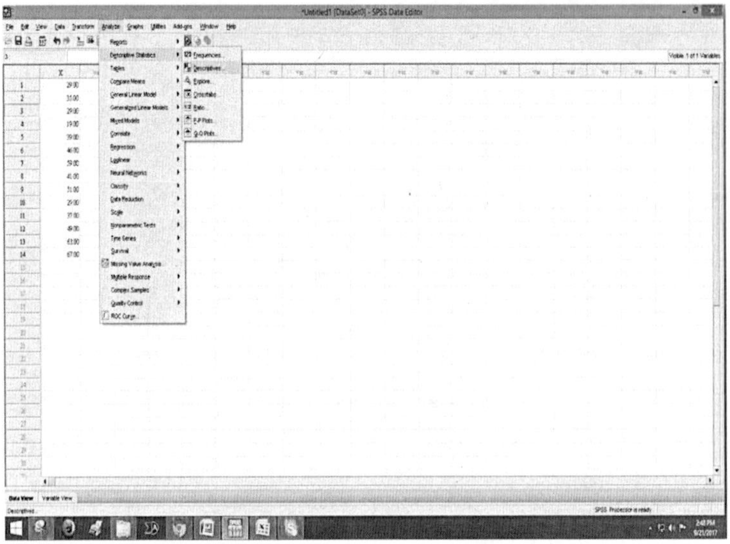

Fig. 1 Selection of the command from the menu.

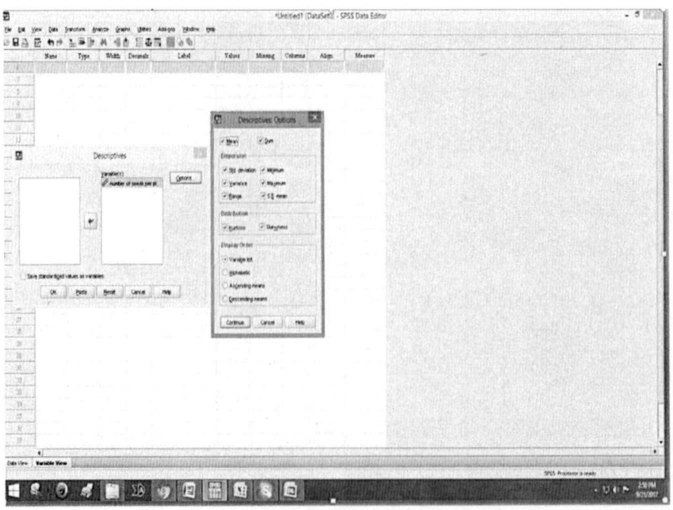

Fig. 2 Selection of the input variable and measures (Options)

Output: Descriptive Statistics: Number of seeds per plant(X)

	N	Range	Minimum	Maximum	Mean		Std. Deviation	Variance
	Statistic	Statistic	Statistic	Statistic	Statistic	Std. Error	Statistic	Statistic
X	14	48.00	19.00	67.00	42.36	3.79	14.19	201.48
Valid N (listwise)	14							

B. Testing the Normality of the Data

Example: Following data have been obtained on water percentage of a body of 15 fishes of a species. Check whether the data is normal.

X: 62 62 63 64 67 68 71 72 71 69 68 64 66 68

SPSS Commands (Step by Step)

Analyze, Explore, Put X in Dependent, Click Plots, Normality Plots, Continue and OK.

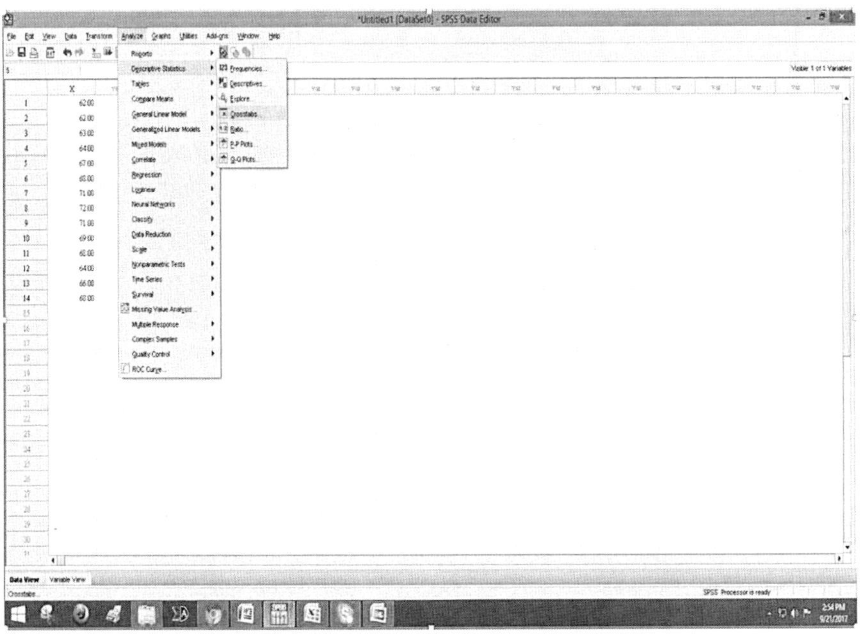

Fig. 3 Selection of the command (explore) from the menu

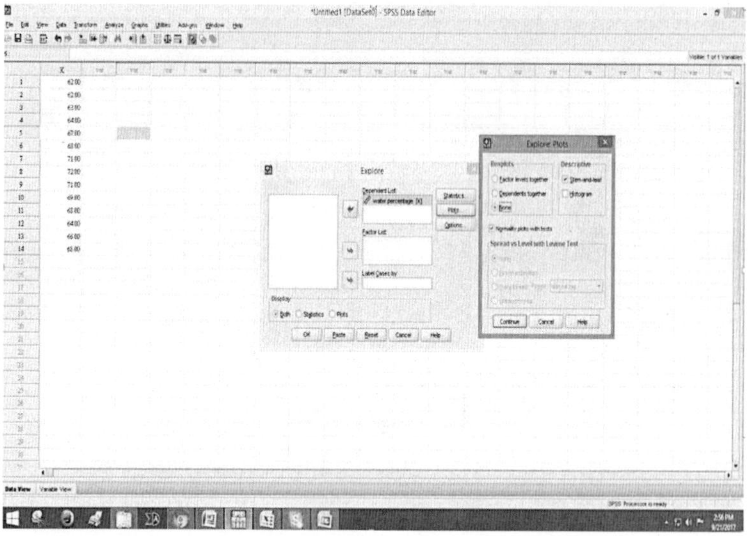

Fig. 4 Selection of the input variable and normality plots with tests

Output: Tests of Normality

	Kolmogorov-Smirnov			Shapiro-Wilk		
	Statistic	df	Sig.	Statistic	df	Sig.
x	.152	14	.200	.934	14	.346

Interpretation: Since p value (Sig.) is >.05, therefore the null hypothesis is accepted. Thus, the data is normal in nature.

C. Correlation

Example: Following table gives the values for the birth weight (X) and the increase in weight between days 70 and 100 of life, expressed as a percentage of the birth weight (Y) for 12 infants.

Y	63	68	75	51	84	114	109	114	39	65	94	93
X	120	104	109	65	89	64	81	116	109	108	93	95

Calculate the coefficient of correlation and interpret the result.

SPSS Commands (Step by Step)

Analyze, Correlate, Bivariate, X and Y, X & Y (Put under variables), Pearson correlation, and OK.

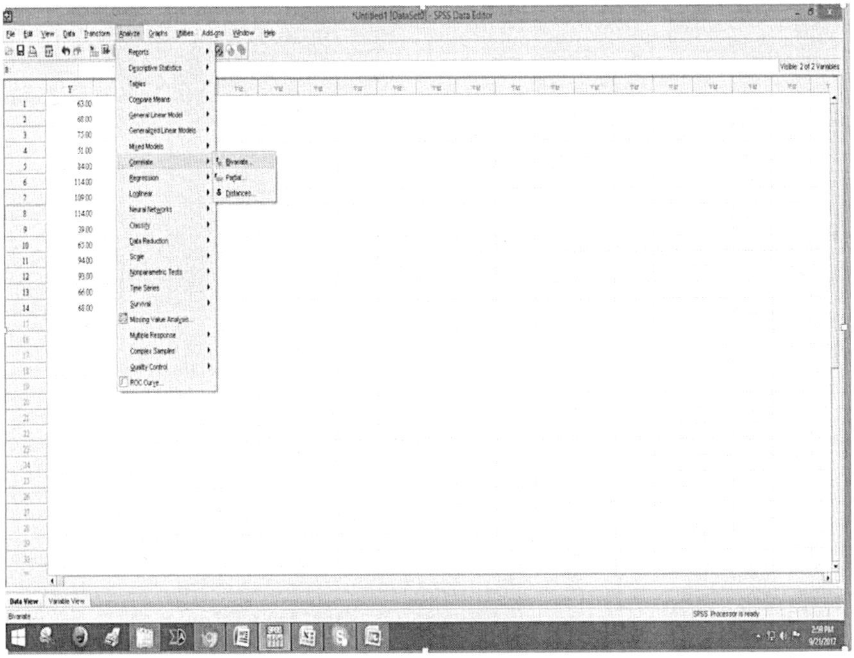

Fig. 5 Selection of the command (correlation bivariate) from the menu

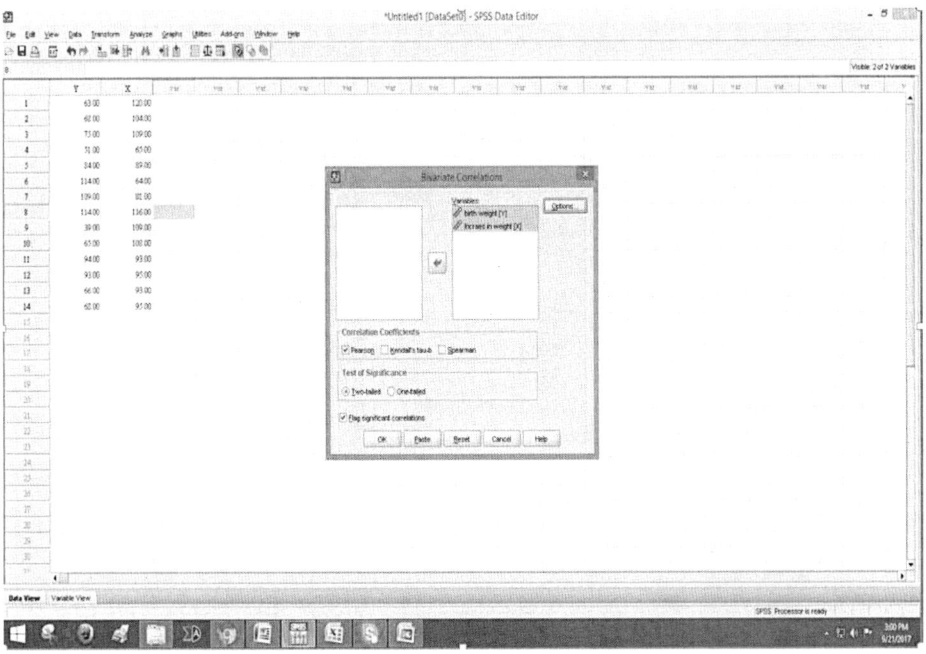

Fig. 6 Selection of the input variable and correlation option

Output: Correlations

Y	X		
Y	Pearson Correlation	1	-.259
	Sig. (2-tailed)		.416
	N	12	12
X	Pearson Correlation	-.259	1
	Sig. (2-tailed)	.416	
	N	12	12

Interpretation: Here, p-value = 0.416 indicates that the correlation coefficient r = -0.259 is insignificant. Thus, we conclude that the birth weight is not significantly correlated with the increase in weight between days 70 and 100 of life.

D. Regression (Linear & Multiple)

Example: Following is the data on keeping quality of milk samples(y), Methylene Blue Reduction time(x_1) and logarithm of standard plate count (x_2) obtained in a study of bacteriological quality of milk.

y	26.0	32.0	32.0	12.0	10.0	10.0	26.0	10.0	24.0	22.0	22.0	20.0	22.0	18.0	22.0
x_1	16.0	16.0	24.0	2.0	6.0	2.0	22.0	3.0	13.0	2.0	4.0	14.0	4.0	22.0	16.0
x_2	5.3	4.2	5.5	4.6	5.1	5.3	4.8	5.0	5.2	7.4	6.5	6.9	4.7	4.2	6.2
y	20.0	23.0	30.0	22.0	19.0	18.0	17.0	16.0	18.0	16.0	24.0	23.0	24.0	22.0	14.0
x_1	15.0	12.0	13.0	15.0	14.0	16.0	18.0	25.0	23.0	19.0	21.0	23.0	14.0	15.0	13.0
x_2	5.3	6.0	6.2	7.5	3.6	4.6	6.0	4.3	5.8	5.6	4.2	4.7	6.5	5.3	4.6

a) Fit the **Simple linear regression** equation of y on x_1.

SPSS Commands (Step by Step) for Simple Linear regression

Analyze, Regression, Linear, Y (Put under Dependent), x_1 (Put under Independent) and OK.

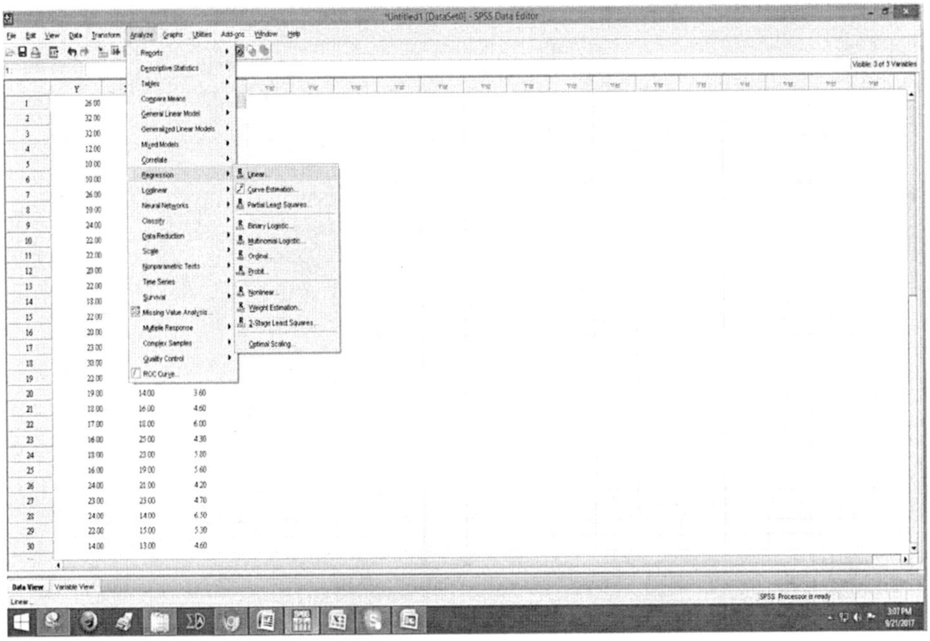

Fig. 7 Selection of the command (Regression linear) from the menu

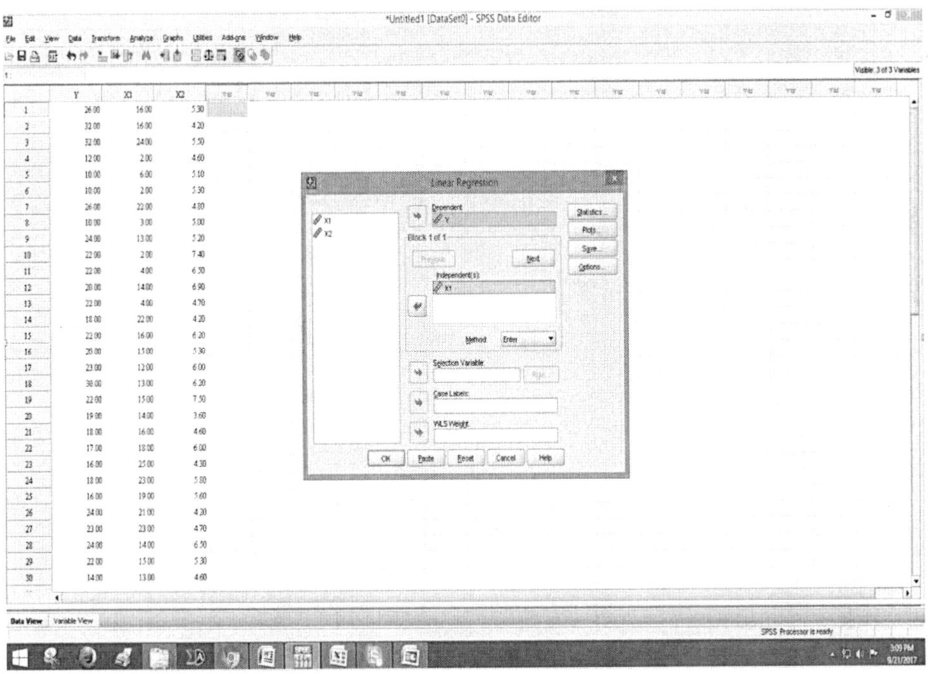

Fig. 8 Selection of the input variables dependent and independent

Output:

Model Summary

Model	R	R Square	Adjusted R Square	Std. Error of the Estimate
1	.400[a]	**.160**	.130	5.47021

ANOVA

Model		Sum of Squares	df	Mean Square	F	Sig.
1	Regression	159.616	1	159.616	5.334	**.029**[a]
	Residual	837.851	28	29.923		
	Total	997.467	29			

Coefficients

Model		Unstandardized Coefficients		Standardized Coefficients	t	Sig.
		B	Std. Error	Beta		
1	(Constant)	**15.790**	2.258		6.993	.000
	X1	**.332**	.144	.400	2.310	.029

b) Fit the **Multiple Regression Analysis** y versus x_1 and x_2.

SPSS Commands (Step by Step) Multiple Linear regression

Analyze, Regression, Linear, Y (Put under Dependent), x_1 & x_2 (Put under Independent) and OK.

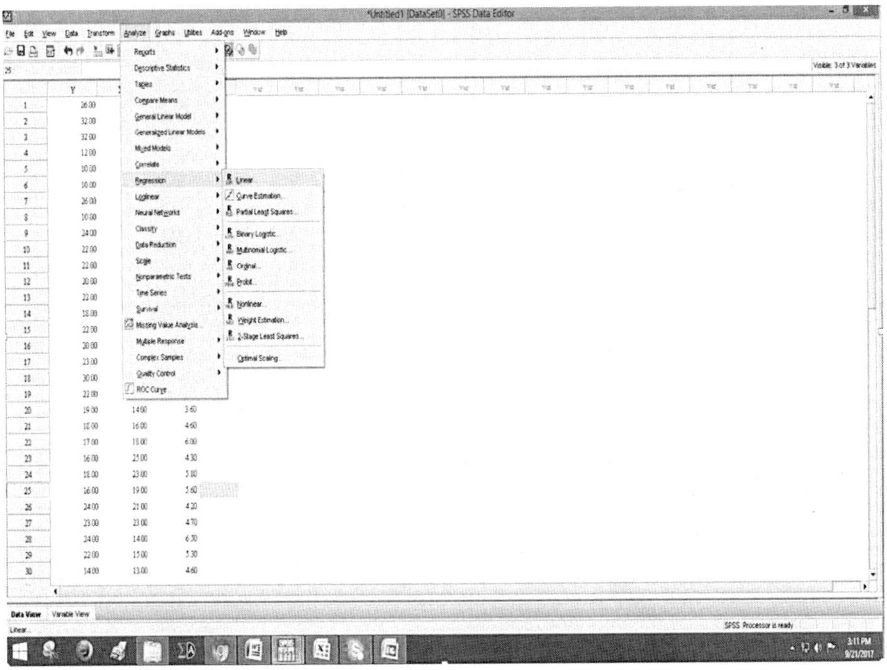

Fig. 9 Selection of the command (Regression linear) from the menu

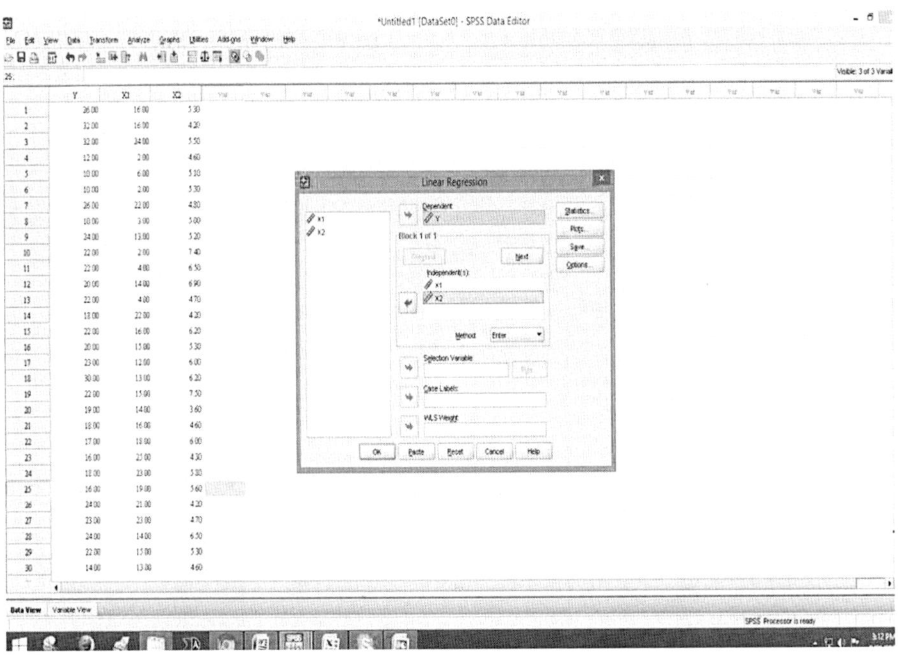

Fig.10 Selection of the input variables Y and X_1& X_2 (independent)

Output:

Model Summary

Model	R	R Square	Adjusted R Square	Std. Error of the Estimate
1	.471[a]	.222	.164	5.36252

a) Predictors: (Constant), X2, X1

ANOVA

Model		Sum of Squares	df	Mean Square	F	Sig.
1	Regression	221.038	2	110.519	3.843	.034[a]
	Residual	776.429	27	28.757		
	Total	997.467	29			

b) Predictors: (Constant), X2, X1

Coefficients

Model		Unstandardized Coefficients		Standardized Coefficients	t	Sig.
		B	Std. Error	Beta		
1	(Constant)	6.909[ns]	6.467		1.068	.295
	X1	.381[*]	.145	.459	2.630	.014
	X2	1.530[ns]	1.047	.255	1.461	.155

* Significant at 5 percent level and ns means non significant

Interpretation

a) In case of simple linear regression the F value of ANOVA is 5.334 (p-value=0.029), which indicates the model is significant and the independent variable can be used to study the Y. Further, R^2 = 0.16 i.e. 16 percent variation of the Y can be explained by the variable X. The regression equation is $Y= 15.79^{**}+ .322X_1^{*}$, which implies that if X_1 increases by one unit then increase in Y i.e. the quality of milk by 0.322 unit from the average level of Y.

b) In case of multiple linear regression, the F value of ANOVA is 3.843 (p-value=0.034), which indicates the model is significant and the independent variables(X_1& X_2) can be used to study the Y. Further, R^2 = 0.222 i.e. 22.2 percent variation of the Y can be explained by the variables X_1& X_2. Further, the regression equation is $Y = 6.909^{ns} + 0.381X_1^{*} + 1.530X_2^{ns}$.In this equation, the value $b_{yx1.x2} = 0.381$ means that on the average, the quality of milk samples increases by 0.381 units if the Methylene blue reduction time is increased by one unit, eliminating the linear effect of the standard plate count.

Testing of Hypothesis

1. One Sample t-test

Example: The average number of stray dogs in an area for the past 50 years was found to be 106. Over the last 10 years the counts have been recorded in the table below.

Year	2005	2006	2007	2008	2009	2010	2011	2012	2013	2014
Dogs count	108	131	156	113	105	99	140	123	110	133

Test whether there been a change in the number of stray dogs to 100 in the area?

SPSS Commands (Step by Step)

Analyze, Compare means, One sample t-test, Y (Put under test variables) and OK.

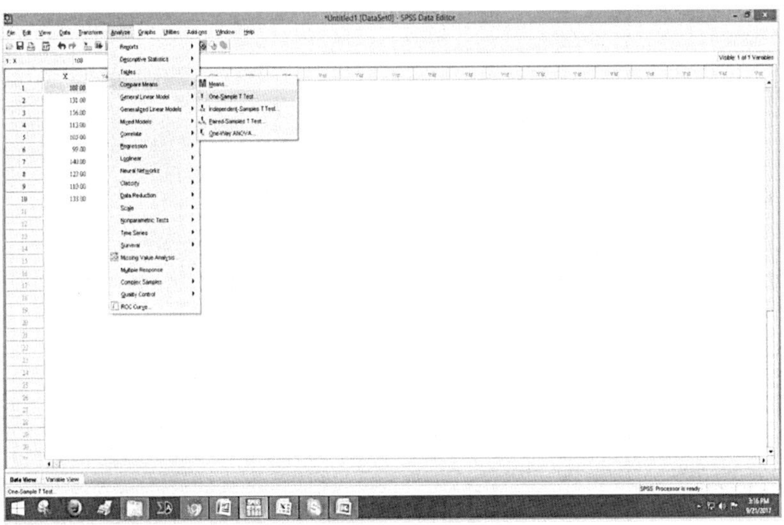

Fig. 11 Selection of the command (compare means and one sample) from the menu

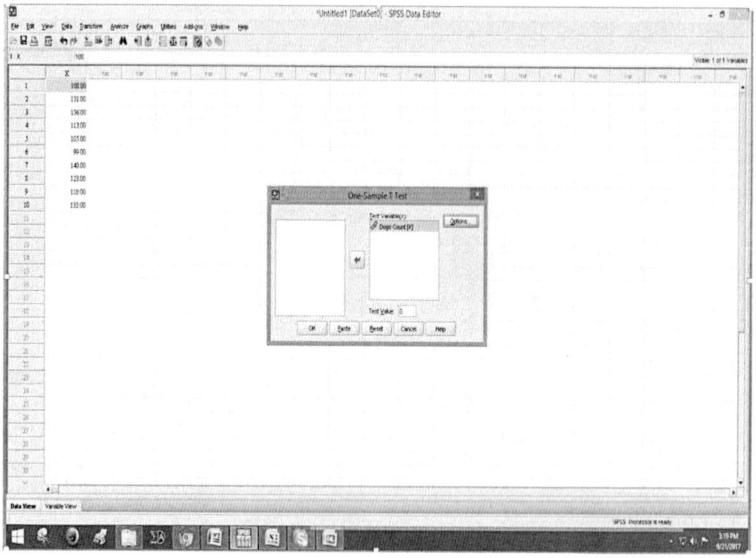

Fig. 12 Selection of the test variable and test value

Output: One-Sample Statistics

	N	Mean	Std. Deviation	Std. Error Mean
dogs count	10	1.2180E2	18.01728	5.69756

	Test Value = 100					
	t	df	Sig. (2-tailed)	Mean Difference	95% Confidence Interval of the Difference	
					Lower	Upper
dogs count	3.826	9	.004	21.80000	8.9112	34.6888

Interpretation: Here, the **p value** of t test is less than 0.05 indicating that there is no change in the number of stray dogs equal to 100 in the area.

2. Two sample t-test (Independent Samples)

Example: A study of the effect of caffeine on muscle metabolism used eighteen male volunteers who each underwent. Nine of the men were randomly selected to take a capsule containing pure caffeine one hour before the test. (RER is the ratio of CO_2 produced to

O_2 consumed and is an indicator of whether energy is being obtained from carbohydrates or fats).Experimenter wanted to check whether, on average, caffeine changes RER. The two populations *i.e.,* "men who have not taken caffeine" and "men who have taken caffeine" have been considered for arm exercise tests. During each exercise the subject's respiratory exchange ratio (RER) was measured. The obtained were:

RER(%)

Men who have not taken caffeine	Men who have taken caffeine
105	96
119	99
100	94
97	89
96	96
101	93
94	88
95	105
98	88

SPSS Commands (Step by Step)

Analyze, Compare means, Independent- sample t-test, Y (Put under test variables),X(Under grouping variable with coding 1 for **Men who have not taken caffeine** and 2 for **Men who have taken caffeine**) and OK

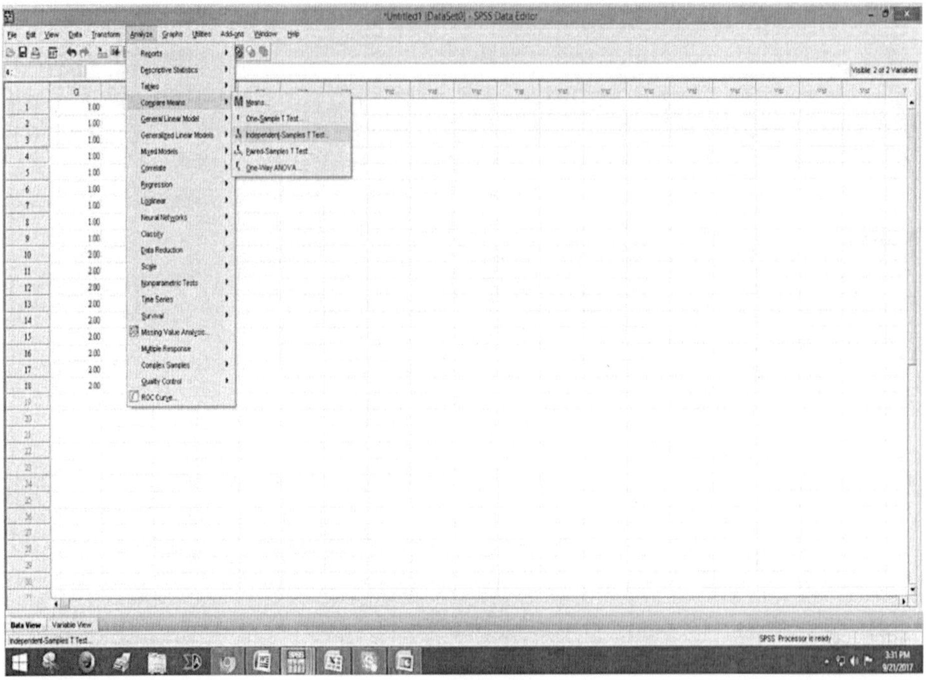

Fig. 13 Selection of the command (compare means & independent sample)

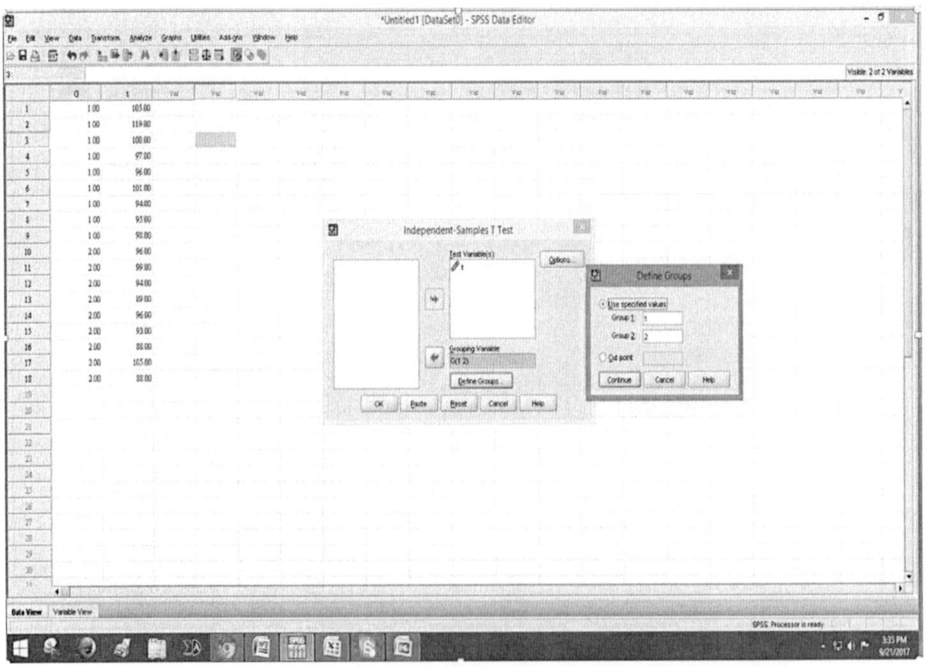

Fig. 14 Selection of the test variable and grouping variable

Output:Group Statistics

Gp	N	Mean	Std. Deviation	Std. Error Mean	
trt	1	9	1.0056E2	7.69921	2.56640
	2	9	94.2222	5.60753	1.86918

Independent Samples Test

	Levene's Test for Equality of Variances		t-test for Equality of Means						
								95% Confidence Interval of the Difference	
	F	Sig.	t	df	Sig. (2-tailed)	Mean Difference	Std. Error Difference	Lower	Upper
trt Equal variances assumed	.197	.663	1.995	16	.063	6.33333	3.17494	-.39724	13.06391
Equal variances not assumed			1.995	14.624	.065	6.33333	3.17494	-.44910	13.11576

Interpretation: It is observed from the output that the p-value of the F-test is more than 0.05. Thus, the test is insignificant means accept the null hypothesis. i.e. the variances of both the groups are equal. Therefore, we will apply the t-test with equal variances otherwise with unequal variances. Further, the p-value of the t-test is more than 0.05 so the test is insignificant means accept the null hypothesis. Thus on average, caffeine does not changes RER.

3. Two sample t-test (Paired t-test or dependent)

Example: The assessment of the stabled horses performing stereotypes (repetitive behaviours indicative of poor welfare: weaving, wind sucking and crib biting) has been done two times to check whether the observation and recording skills had improved each time they watched. The groups' results are displayed in the table below.

First time	Second time
15	52
36	49
59	26
61	65
16	81
36	33
69	74

Test whether there is any change in the behaviour of the horses.

SPSS Commands (Step by Step)

Analyze, Compare means, Paired- sample t-test, Y&X (Put under paired variables) and OK.

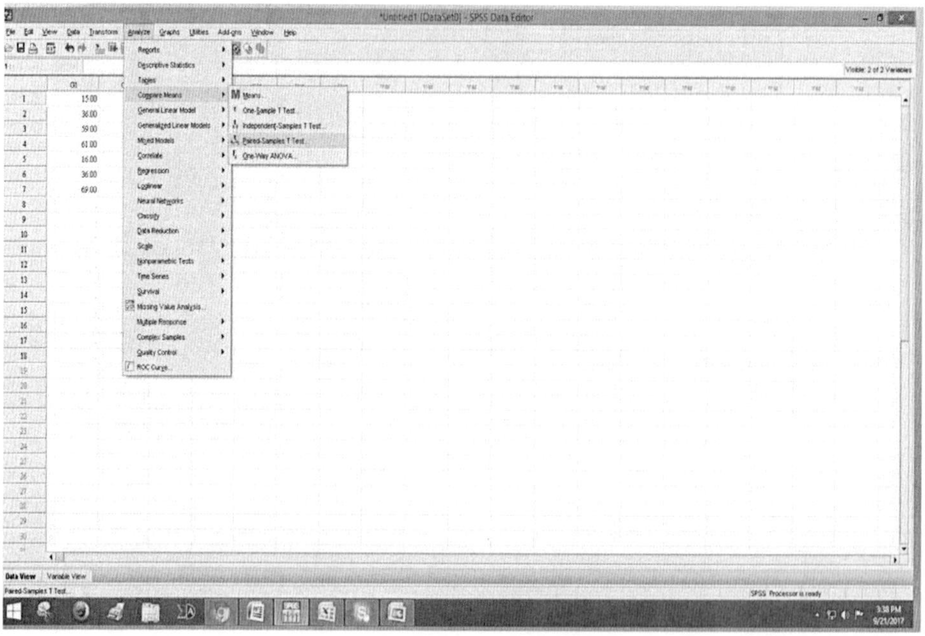

Fig. 15 Selection of the command (paired sample t -test)

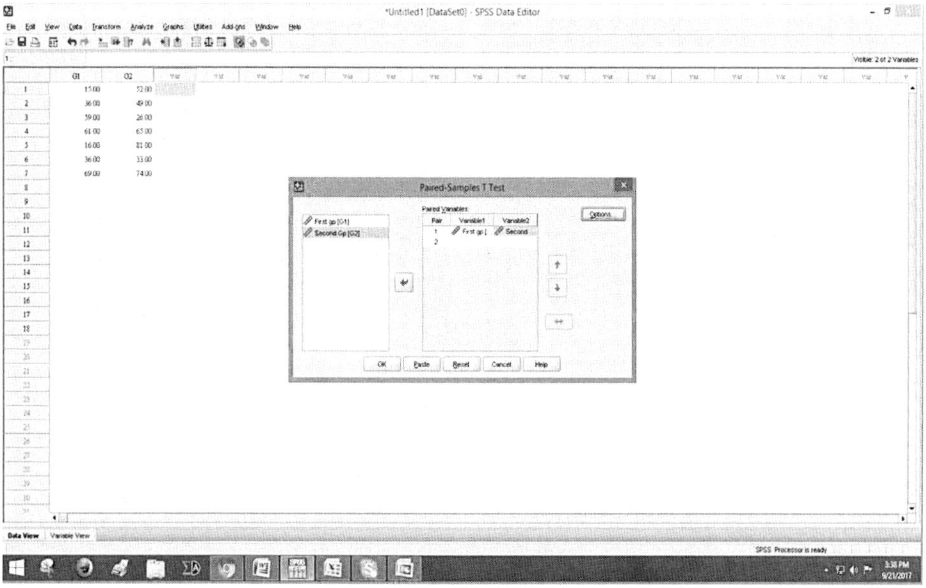

Fig. 16 Selection of the paired variables

Output: Paired Samples Statistics

		Mean	N	Std. Deviation	Std. Error Mean
Pair 1	G1	41.7143	7	21.81524	8.24539
	G2	54.2857	7	20.42641	7.72046

Paired Samples Correlations

	Paired Differences					t	df	Sig. (2-tailed)
				95% C.I. Interval of the Difference				
	Mean	Std. Deviation	Std. Error Mean	Lower	Upper			
Pair 1 G1 - G2	-1.25714E1	31.079	11.747	-41.31	16.172	-1.070	6	0.326

Interpretation: Since $|t_{cal}| < t_{tab}$ (as is clear by P-value > 0.05). Here t is not significant and hence we accept the null hypothesis. We concluded that there is no change in the behaviour of the horse w r t time.

F. CHI SQUARE

A researcher wants to know whether there is a significant difference in two therapies for curing patients of cocaine dependence (defined as not taking cocaine for at least 6 months). He tests 150 patients and obtains the results in the upper left part of the table below (labeled Observed Values).

	Therapy 1	Therapy 2
Cured	31	57
Not Cured	11	51

SPSS Commands (Step by Step): The analysis will be performed in two parts as

i) First: Data, Weight case by T and OK,

ii) Second: Analyze, Descriptive, Crosstab, Shift R to Row, C to Column, Statistics, Chi square, Continue and OK.

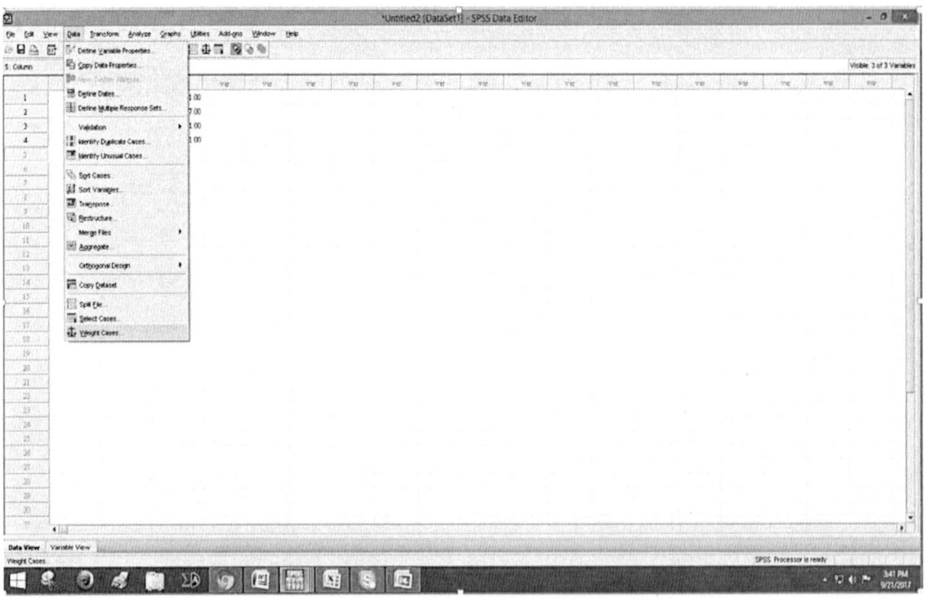

Fig. 17 Insertion of the Data into the Data window

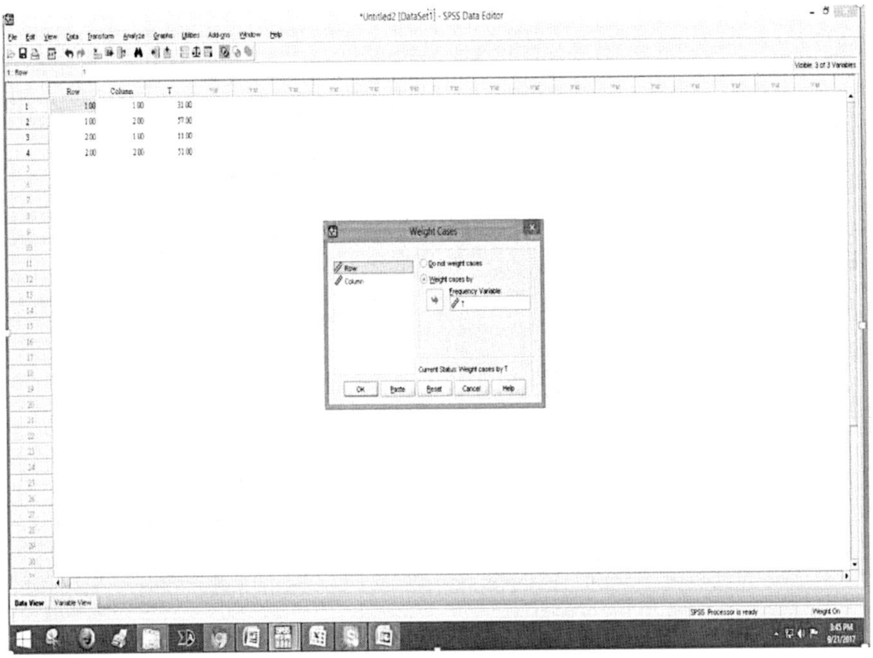

Fig. 18 Assigning weight to the Variable T

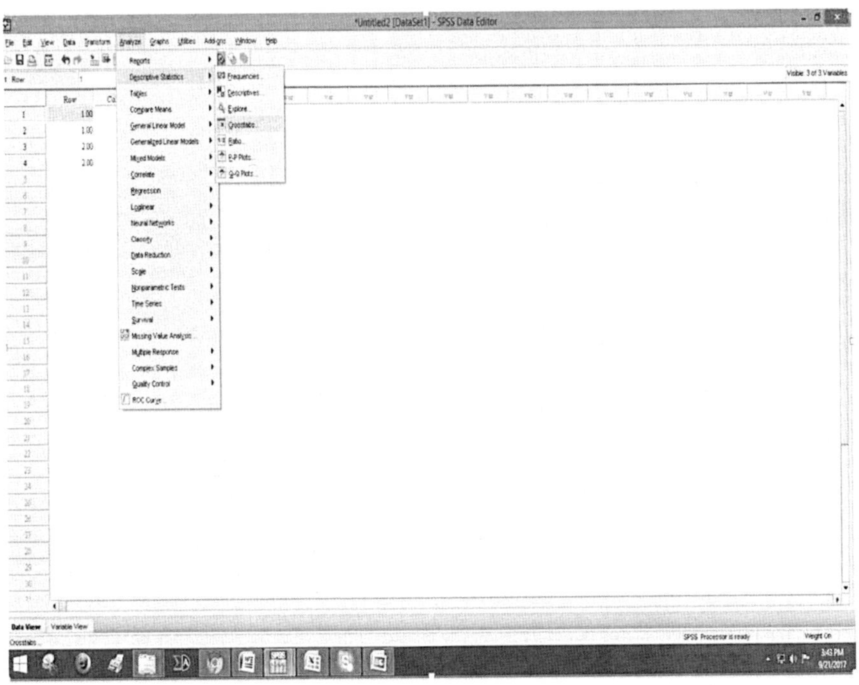

Fig. 19 Selection of the command crosstab (Descriptive statistics)

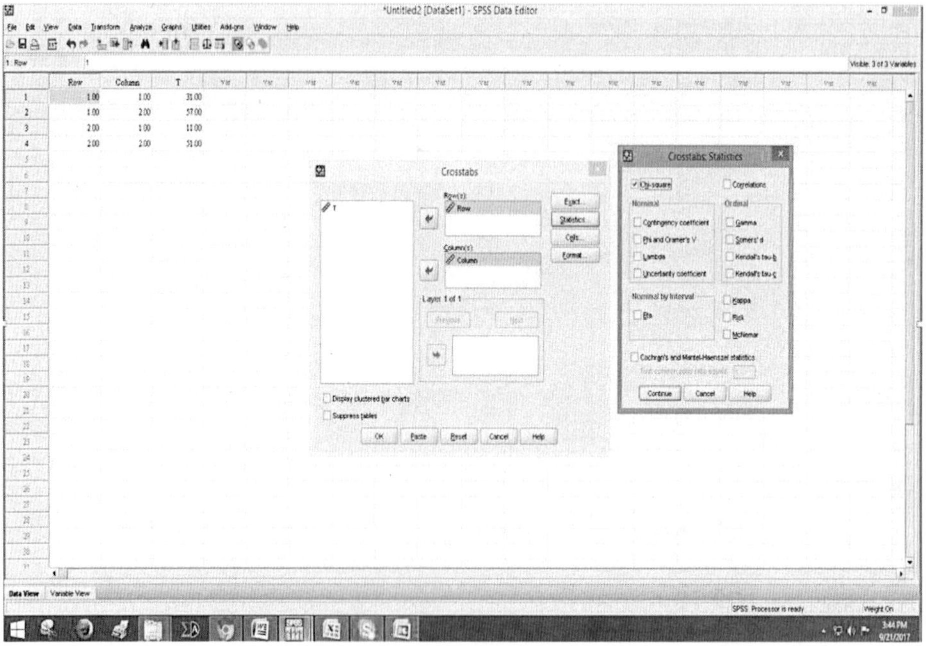

Fig. 20 Selection of the variables and test chi square

Output:

Case Processing Summary

	Cases					
	Valid		Missing		Total	
	N	Percent	N	Percent	N	Percent
R * C	144	100.0%	0	.0%	144	100.0%

R * C Crosstabulation

			C		
			1	2	Total
R	1	Count	31	51	82
		Expected Count	23.9	58.1	82.0
	2	Count	11	51	62
		Expected Count	18.1	43.9	62.0
Total		Count	42	102	144
		Expected Count	42.0	102.0	144.0

Chi-Square Tests

	Value	df	Asymp. Sig. (2-sided)	Exact Sig. (2-sided)	Exact Sig. (1-sided)
Pearson Chi-Square	6.879[a]	1	.009		
Continuity Correction [b]	5.942	1	.015		
Likelihood Ratio	7.134	1	.008		
Fisher's Exact Test				.010	.007
Linear-by-Linear Association	6.831	1	.009		
N of Valid Cases [b]	144				

Interpretation: From the above table; it has been observed that the Pearson chi square value is significant as p- value is less than 0.05. Thus, it can be concluded that the two attributes are not independent.

G. Analysis of Statistical Designs

a) **One way ANOVA**

Example: An experiment was conducted to test 'the effect of 4 dose levels of a drug on kidney weight of Dogs. 4 groups of dogs were taken and one dose level was administrated to each group. After the assigned period, kidney weights were as follows. Kidney weights (X) are expressed as percentage of body weight.

Dose levels			
400 ppm	**200 ppm**	**100 ppm**	**0 ppm**
0.43	0.49	0.34	0.34
0.52	0.48	0.40	0.32
0.43	0.40	0.42	0.33
0.55	0.34	0.40	0.39

Test whether the 4 dose levels have same effect on kidney weight of dogs.

SPSS Commands (Step by Step)

Analyze, Compare means, One-way ANOVA, dose, button (put dose under Dependent list), Treatment (puts treat. Under Factor), Continue, OK

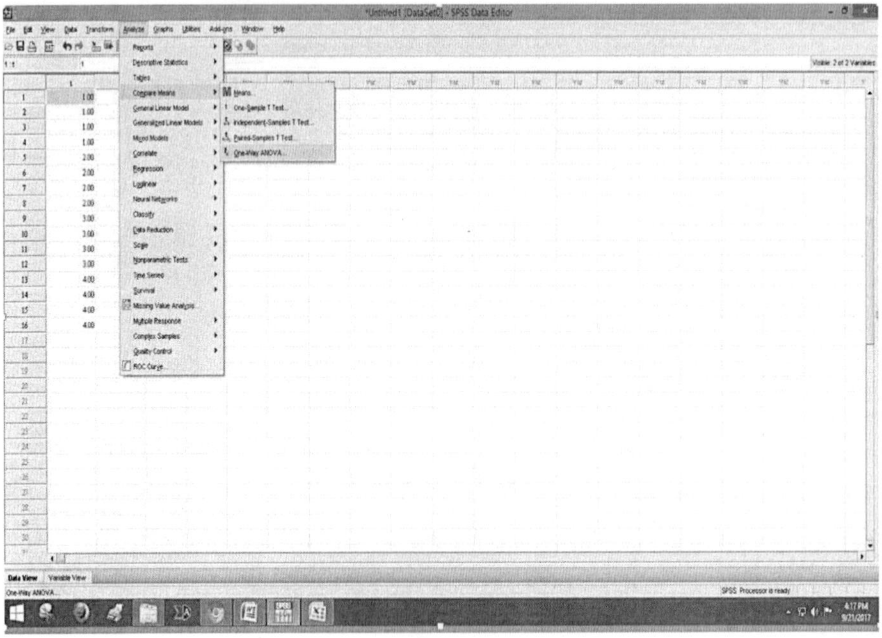

Fig. 21 Selection of the command one way anova in the domain of compare means

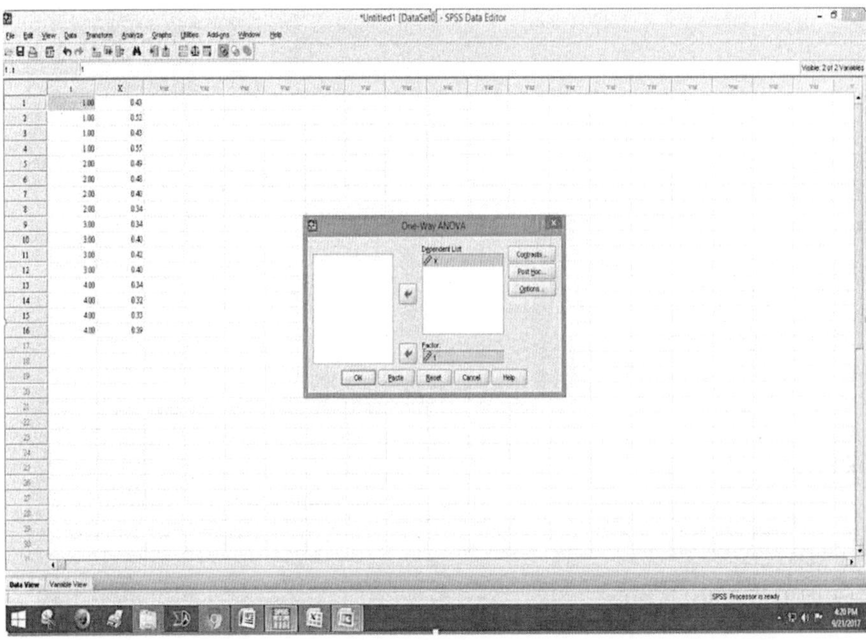

Fig. 22 Shifting of the variables to dependent and factor

Output:

ANOVA

Source of Variation	Sum of Squares	df	Mean Square	F	Sig.
Between Groups	.041	3	.014	4.929	.019
Within Groups	.033	12	.003		
Total Variation	.074	15			

Interpretation

From ANOVA table it has been observed that the dose levels differ significantly (P-value = 0.019) as regards to dose levels of drug. A further comparison among varieties can be made through LSD/CD value.

b) Two Way ANOVA

Following table contains the data on the average daily milk yield of six cows in an experiment on the effect of protein supplement on milk production.

Treatment: A : Protein supplement P_1

B : Protein supplement P_2

C : Protein supplement P_3

Cow Treatment	1	2	3	4	5	6
A	10.4	10.5	5.9	6.7	8	6.7
B	12.6	12.5	11.2	8.8	9.5	12
C	9.5	9.7	12.6	9.1	8.7	10.5

Analyze the data.

SPSS Commands (Step by Step):Analyze, GLM, Milk Yield, button (puts milk yield under Dependent list), Treatment (puts row under Factor, Continue, Model......, Custom, Treatment (puts treatment under model), Continue, OK

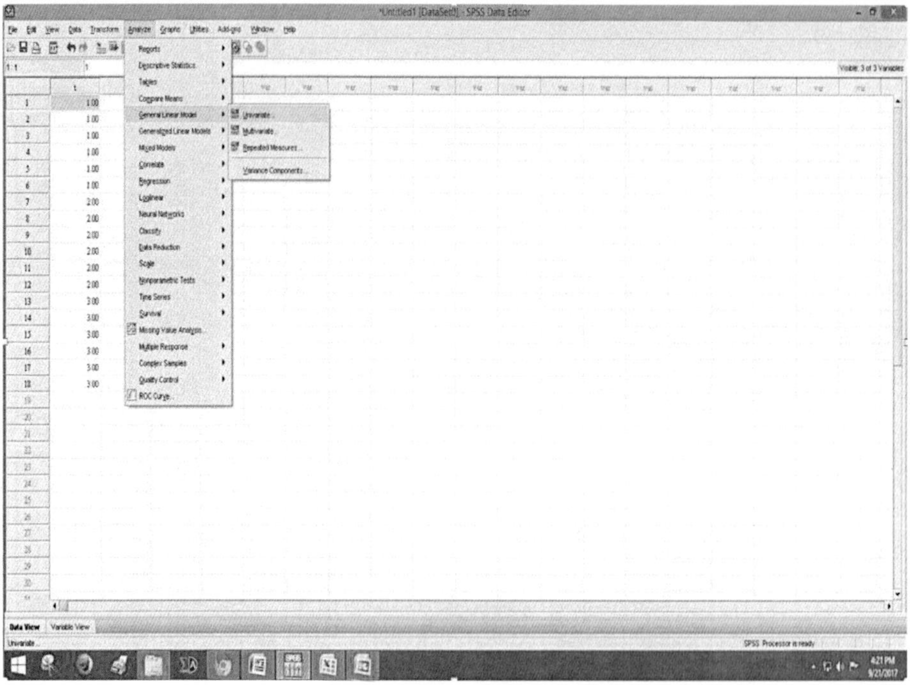

Fig. 23 Selection of the command GLM (univariate)

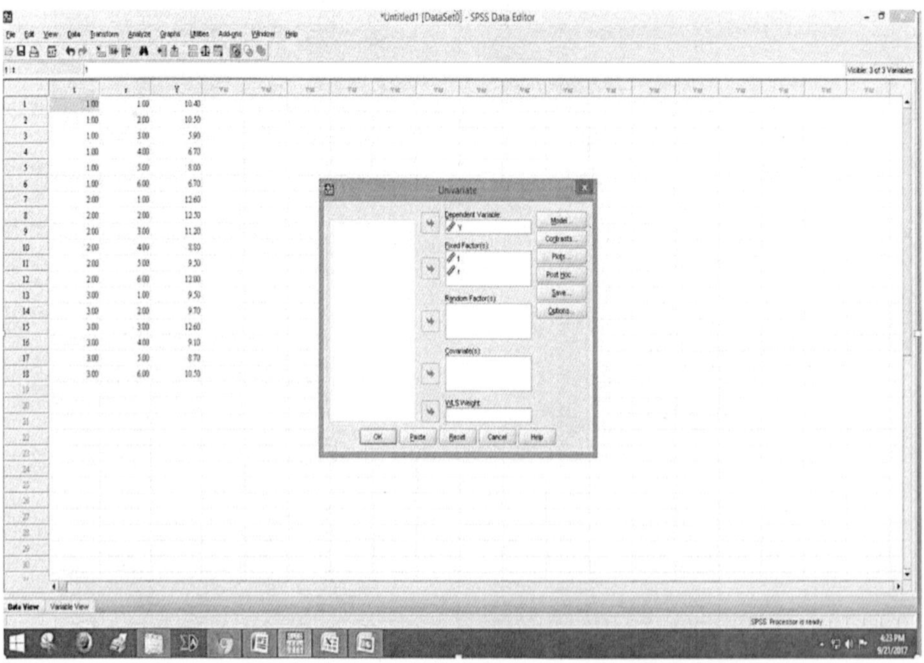

Fig. 24 Shifting of the variables to dependent and factor

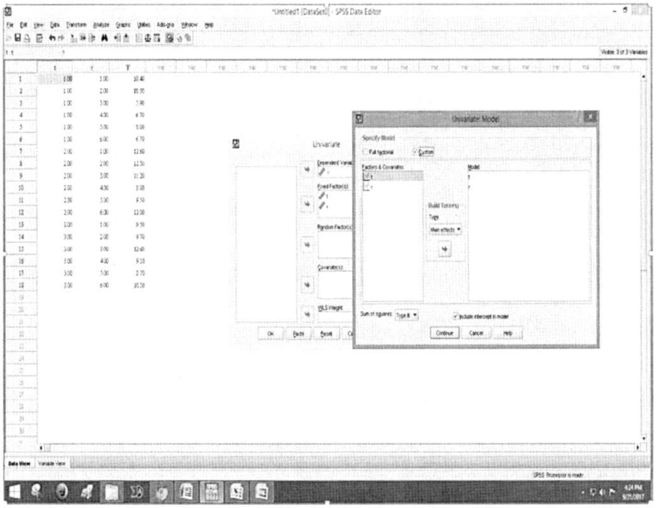

Fig. 25 Selection of the custom model and treatment group

Output: Tests of Between-Subjects Effects

Dependent Variable: Milk yield

Source	Type III Sum of Squares	df	Mean Square	F	Sig.
Corrected Model	46.868[a]	7	6.695	2.713	0.074
Intercept	1699.445	1	1699.445	688.685	0
t	29.023	2	14.512	5.881	0.02
r	17.845	5	3.569	1.446	0.289
Error	24.677	10	2.468		
Total	1770.99	18			
Corrected Total	71.545	17			

a. R Squared = 0.655 (Adjusted R Squared = .414)

Interpretation

From ANOVA table it has been observed that the treatments differ significantly (P-value = 0.020). A further comparison among treatments can be made through LSD/CD value.

c) Three Way ANOVA

Example: Following data have been obtained in latin square design for feeding trail on sheep.

Treatment:

A: Grazing only (control); B Grazing + Maize supplement; C: Grazing + Maize + protein supplement P_1; D: Grazing + Maize + protein supplement P_2; E: Grazing + Maize + protein supplement P_3

D(33)	E(31)	C(29)	B(30)	A(21)
C(48)	D(45)	A(41)	E(45)	B(29)
E(43)	A(29)	B(24)	D(36)	C(35)
B(40	C(35)	E(43)	A(23)	D(31)
A(26)	B(24)	D(26)	C(33)	E(26)

Analyze the data.

SPSS Commands (Step to Step)

Analyze, GLM, Yield, button (puts yield under Dependent list), Row (puts row under Factor), Column, Treatment, Continue, Model……, Custom, Row (puts row under model), Column, Treatment (puts column and treatment under model), Continue, OK

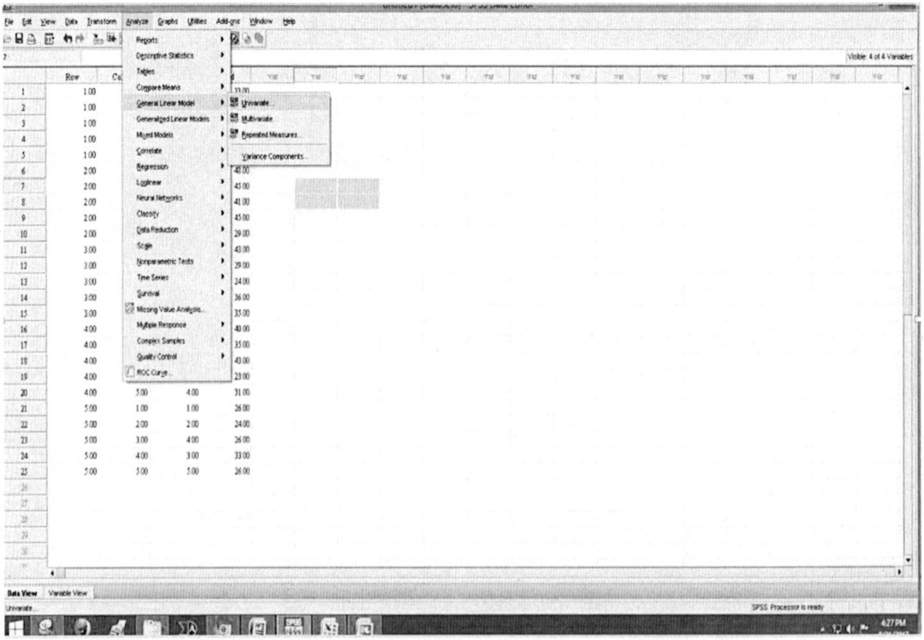

Fig. 26 Selection of the command GLM (univariate) for three way

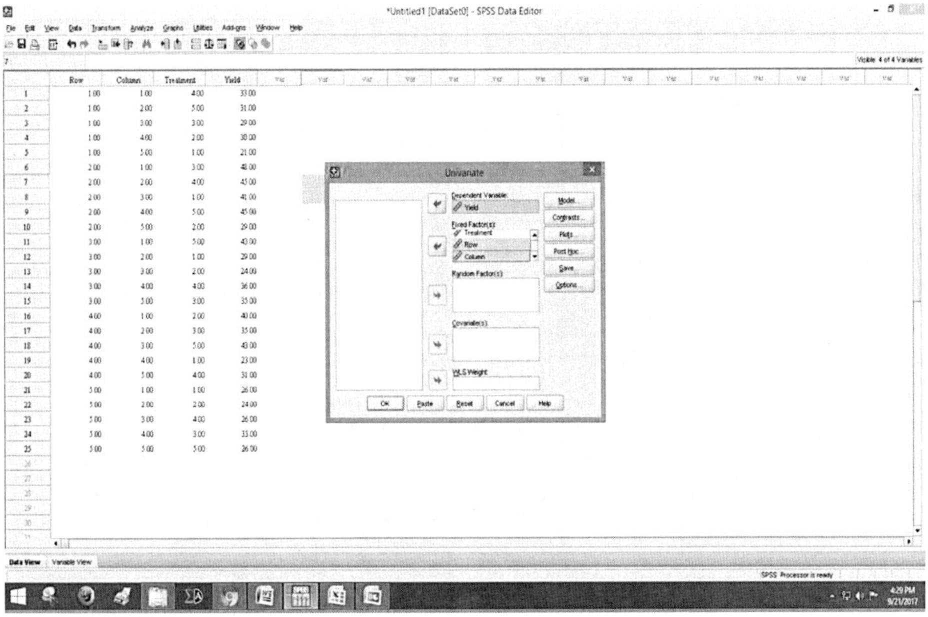

Fig. 27 Shifting of the variables to dependent and factor

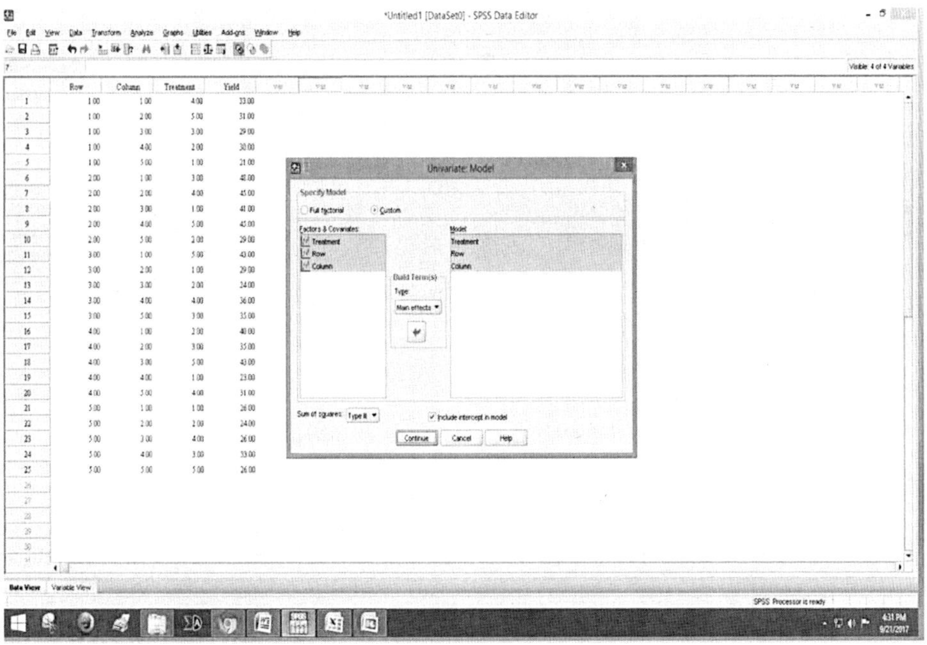

Fig. 28 Selection of the custom model and treatment group

Output:

Tests of Between-Subjects Effects

Dependent Variable: y

Source	Type III Sum of Squares	df	Mean Square	F	Sig.
Corrected Model	1228.880[a]	12	102.407	5.295	.004
Intercept	27291.040	1	27291.040	1.411E3	.000
r	648.560	4	162.140	8.384	.002
c	232.560	4	58.140	3.006	.062
t	347.760	4	86.940	4.495	.019
Error	232.080	12	19.340		
Total	28752.000	25			
Corrected Total	1460.960	24			

a. R Squared = .841 (Adjusted R Squared = .682)

Interpretation

From ANOVA table we obtain that the treatments differ significantly (P-value = 0.019). A further comparison among treatments can be made through multiple comparisons test.

References

Ajai S. Gaur & Sanjaya S. Gaur (2009). Statistical Methods for Practice and Research: a guide to Data analysis Using SPSS. Sage Publications Inc.

L. S. Aiken and S.G. West (1999). Multiple Regression: testing and Interpreting Interactions. Newbury Park, CA: Sage Publications

Manish Kumar Sharma, Anil Bhat and M I J Bhat. (2017). Computer in Agriculture: Fundamentals and research. New India Publishing Agency.

Ramez Elamseri, (2008). Fundamental of Database Systems, Pearson Education India.

V.N. Amble. (1975). Statistical M ethods in Animal Sciences. Indian Society of Agricultural Statistics, New Delhi.

❑❑❑

Chapter 4

Retrieval of Sequences, Multiple Sequence Alignment, Detection and Annotation of SNP's

Nishant Kumar, Nusrat Nabi Khan, Dibyendu Chakraborty and Dhirendra Kumar and Vikas Mahajan

A structured set of data held in computer especially one that is accessible in various ways. Database search and retrieval means obtaining data from available database. In order to retrieve the desired data the user present a set of criteria by a query.

There are several reasons to search databases. One of which is when obtaining a new DNA sequence, one needs to know whether it has already been deposited in the databanks, or whether they contain any homologous sequences. Given a putative coding ORF, we can search for homologous proteins. One can also use data base to find similar non-coding DNA stretches in the database like repeat elements or regulatory sequences for instance. There are other uses for specific purpose, like locating false priming sites for a set of PCR oligonucleotides.

There are different databases available for nucleotide and protein sequences. Examples of nucleotide databases are.

1. The large databases: Genbank (US), Embl (Europe), DDBJ (Japan).
2. Genomic databases: Human (GDB), mouse (MGB), yeast (SGB), etc.
3. Special databases: ESTs (expressed sequence tags), STSs (sequence-tagged sites), EPD(eukaryotic promotor database), REPBASE (repetitive sequence database) and the examples of protein databases.

4. The large databases are: Swiss-Prot (high level of annotation), PIR (protein identification resource).
5. Translated databases, like SPTREMBL (translated EMBL), GenPept (translation of coding regions in GenBank).
6. Special databases, like PDB (sequences derived from the 3D structure BrookhavenPDB).

How to Perform Database-Searching

There are three data retrieval systems of particular relevance to molecular biologist: Sequence Retrieval System (SRS), Entrez, DBGET. These systems allow text searching of multiple molecular biology databases and provide links to relevant information for entries that match the search criteria.

A. Sequence Retrieval System (SRS)

It is a homogeneous interface to over 80 biological databases that had been developed at the European Bioinformatics Institute (EBI) at Hinxton, UK. It includes databases of sequences, metabolic pathways, transcription factors, application results (like BLAST, SSEARCH, FASTA), protein 3D structures, genomes, mappings, mutations, and locus specific mutations. The web page listing all the databases contains a link to a description page about the database including the date on which it was last updated.

a) **Entrez**

It is a molecular biology database and retrieval system. Developed by the National Center for Biotechnology information (NCBI). It is entry point for exploring distinct but integrated databases. Of the three text-based database systems, Entrez is the easiest to use, but also offers more limited information to search.

b) **DBGET**

It is an integrated database retrieval system, developed at the university of Tokyo provided access to 20 databases, one at a time. Having more limited options, the DBGET is less recommended than the two others.

Main Algorithms for Database Searching

There are three main search tools: FastA, BLAST and SW-search. BLAST - Basic Local Alignment Search Tool.

Blast programs use a heuristic search algorithm. The programs use the statistical methods of Karlin and Altschul. Blast programs were designed for fast database searching, with minimal sacrifice of sensitivity for distantly related sequences. The programs search databases in a special compressed format.

Some of the Variants of BLAST are BLASTN, BLASTP, BLASTX, TBLASTN, and TBLAST. The program compares the query to each sequence in database using heuristic rules to speed up the pair wise comparison. It creates sequence abstraction by listing exact and similar words. This is done in advance for each sequence in the data base on the run for a certain query. BLAST finds similar words between the query and each database sequence. It then extends such words to obtain high scoring sequence pairs (HSPs). It also calculates statistics analytically like FastA does. BLAST output is very similar to the FASTA output. It contains information for each hit (Including hit name, description, length), score of hit (how many identical residues, how many residues contributing positively to the score, and the statistics of the score), and the local alignment itself.

Multiple sequence alignment

Multiple nucleotide or amino acid sequence alignment techniques are usually done for characterization of protein families, or identification of shared regions of homology in a multiple sequence. It is also done for the determination of the consensus sequence of several aligned sequences. It helps in predicting the secondary and tertiary structures of new sequences. It is also used in preliminary step in molecular evolution analysis using and for constructing phylogenetic trees.

The algorithm of multiple alignments is as follows. First it Perform all pairwise comparisons between the sequences. Then it performs cluster analysis on the pairwise data to generate a cluster hierarchy. This hierarchy may build in the form of a binary tree or a simple ordering. Finally it construct the multiple alignment by first aligning the most similar pair of sequences, then the next most similar pair and so on. Once an alignment of two sequences has been made, it remains fixed. Thus for a set of sequences A, B, C, D having aligned A with C and B with D the alignment of A, B, C, D is obtained by comparing the alignment of A and C with that of B and D using averaged scores at each aligned position.

Clustal W is a general purpose multiple alignment program for DNA or proteins. Clustal W improves the sensitivity of progressive multiple sequence alignment through sequence weighting, positions specific gap penalties and weight matrix choice. It can create multiple alignments, manipulate existing alignments, perform profile analysis and create phylogenetic trees. Alignment can be constructed either slow but accurate or by fast but more approximated.

Single nucleotide polymorphisms

Single nucleotide polymorphisms or SNPs (pronounced "snips") are DNA sequence variations that occur when a single nucleotide (A, T, C, or G) in the genome sequence is altered. For example a SNP might change the DNA sequence AAGGCTAA to ATGGCTAA. For a variation to be considered a SNP, it must occur in at least 1% of the population. SNPs, which make up about 90% of all human genetic variation, occur every 100 to 300 bases along the 3 billion-base human genome. Two of every three SNPs involve the replacement of cytosine (C) with thymine (T). SNPs can occur in both coding (gene) and noncoding regions of the genome. Although more than 99% of human DNA sequences are the same across the population, variations in DNA sequence can have a major impact on how humans respond to disease like infection of bacteria and viruses, exposure to toxins and chemicals and drugs and other therapies. SNPs are also evolutionarily stable not changing much from generation to generation making them easier to follow in population studies.

There are several methods of detection of SNP like RFLP, Denaturing gradient gel electrophporesis, Single Strand Conformation Polymorphism (SSCP), Mismatch Repair Detection (MRD), Heteroduplex Analysis (HA), Denaturing High Performance Liquid Chromatography, UNG-Mediated T-Sequencing, Sequencing by Hybridization and Direct DNA Sequencing.

□□□

Chapter 5

Phylogenetic Tree and its Analysis

Nishant Kumar, Nusrat Nabi Khan, Dibyendu Chakraborty and Dhirendra Kumar

A phylogenetic tree or evolutionary tree is a branching diagram or tree showing the inferred evolutionary relationships among various biological species or other entities, their phylogeny based upon similarities and differences in their physical or genetic characteristics.

Understanding a phylogeny is a lot like reading a family tree. The root of the tree represents the ancestral lineage, and the tips of the branches represent the descendants of that ancestor. As you move from the root to the tips, you are moving forward in time.

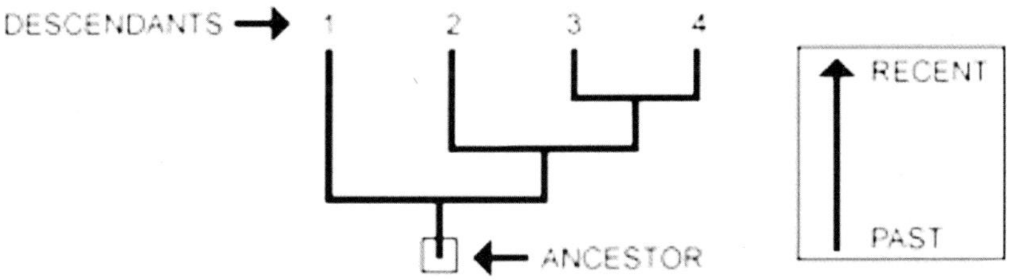

When a lineage splits (speciation), it is represented as branching on a phylogeny. When a speciation event occurs, a single ancestral lineage gives rise to two or more daughter lineages.

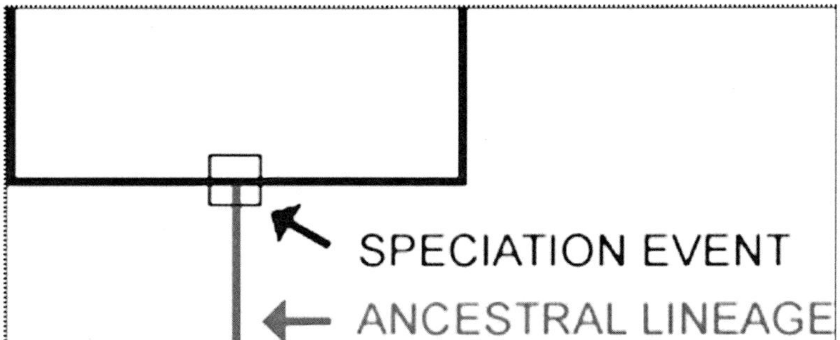

Phylogenies trace patterns of shared ancestry between lineages. Each lineage has a part of its history that is unique to it alone and parts that are shared with other lineages.

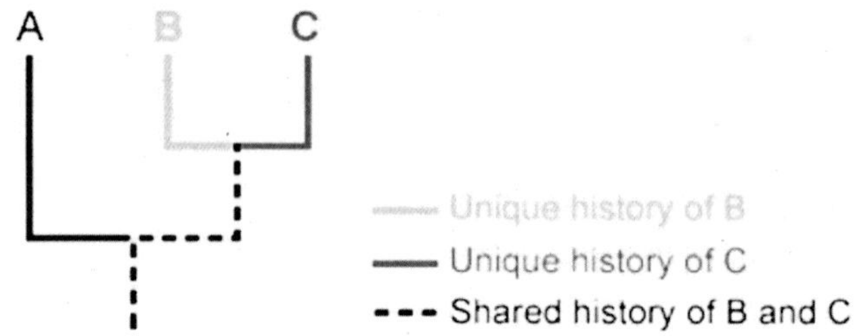

Similarly, each lineage has ancestors that are unique to that lineage and ancestors that are shared with other lineages ie common ancestors

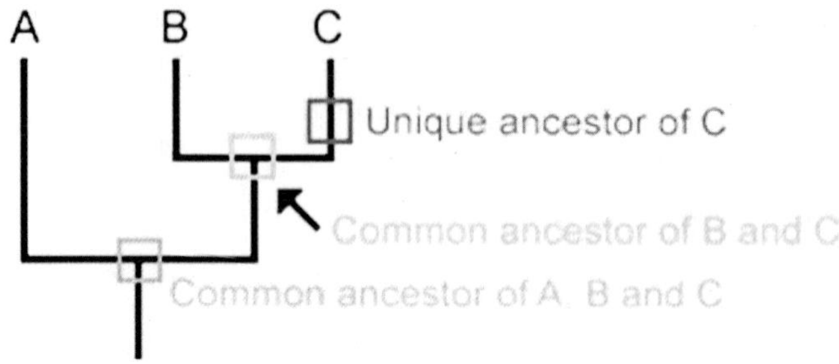

A clade is a grouping that includes a common ancestor and all the descendants (living and extinct) of that ancestor. Using a phylogeny, it is easy to tell if a group of lineages forms a clade.

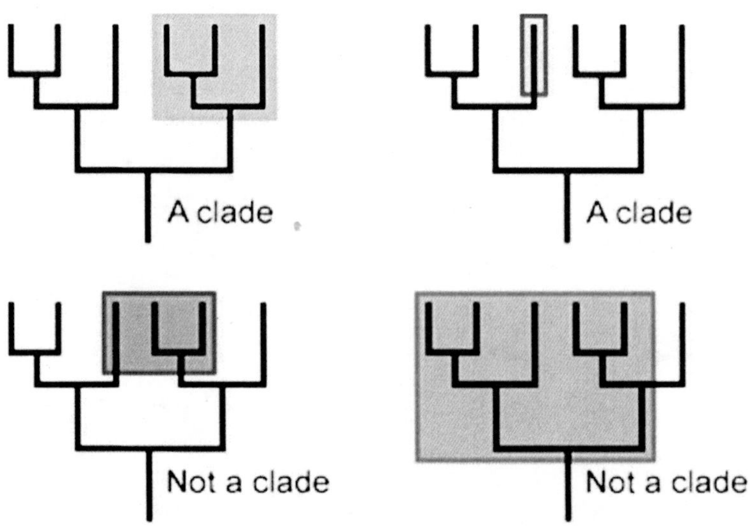

Clades are nested within one another *i.e.* they form a nested hierarchy. A clade may include many thousands of species or just a few.

The tips of a phylogeny represent descendent lineages. Depending on how many branches of the tree you are including however, the descendants at the tips might be different populations of a species, different species, or different clades, each composed of many species.

Several times in the past, biologists have committed themselves to the erroneous idea that life can be organized on a ladder of lower to higher organisms. This idea lies at the heart of Aristotle's Great Chain of Being. Similarly, it's easy to misinterpret phylogenies as implying that some organisms are more advanced than others, however, phylogenies don't imply this at all.

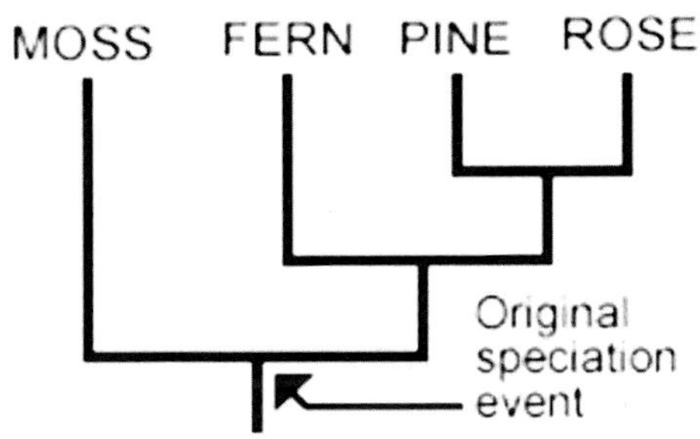

In this highly simplified phylogeny, a speciation event occurred resulting in two lineages. One led to the mosses of today, the other led to the fern, pine, and rose. Since that speciation event, both lineages have had an equal amount of time to evolve. So, although mosses branch off early on the tree of life and share many features with the ancestor of all land plants, living moss species are not ancestral to other land plants. Nor are they more primitive. Mosses are the cousins of other land plants.

So when reading a phylogeny, it is important to keep three things in mind:

1. Evolution produces a pattern of relationships among lineages that is tree like, not ladder-like.

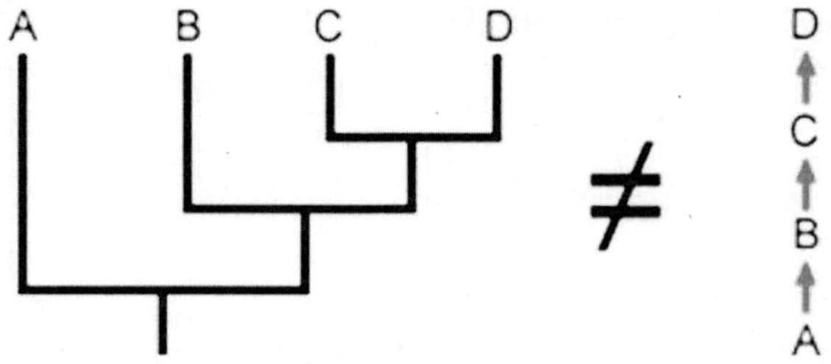

2. Just because we tend to read phylogenies from left to right, there is no correlation with level of advancement.

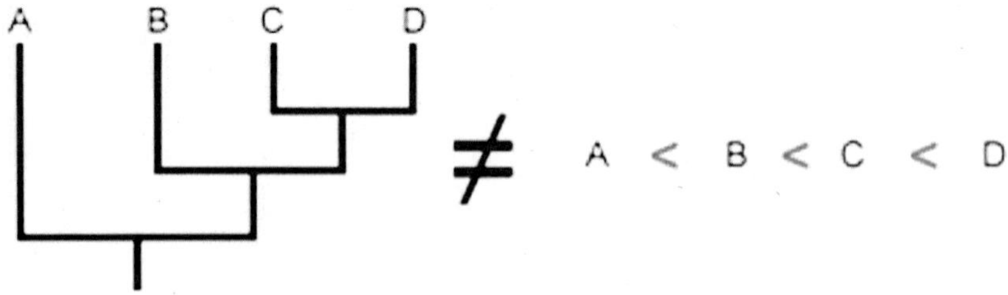

3. For any speciation event on a phylogeny, the choice of which lineage goes to the right and which goes to the left is arbitrary. The following phylogenies are equivalent:

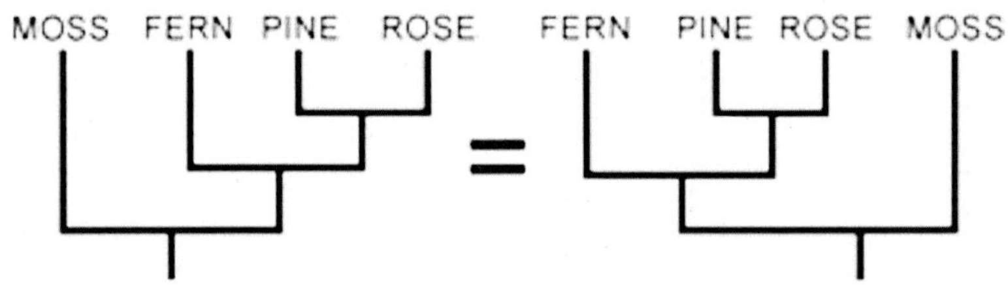

Molecular Phylogeny is the branch of phylogeny that analyses hereditary molecular differences, mainly in DNA sequences, to gain information on an organism's evolutionary relationships. The result of a molecular phylogenetic analysis is expressed in a phylogenetic tree. Molecular phylogenetics is one aspect of molecular systematics, a broader term that also includes the use of molecular data in taxonomy and biogeography.

Every living organism contains DNA, RNA, and proteins. In general, closely related organisms have a high degree of agreement in the molecular structure of these substances, while the molecules of organisms distantly related usually show a pattern of dissimilarity. Conserved sequences, such as mitochondrial DNA, are expected to accumulate mutations over time, and assuming a constant rate of mutation, and provides a molecular clock for dating divergence. Molecular phylogeny uses such data to build a "relationship tree" that shows the probable evolution of various organisms. High throughput sequencing may also be used to obtain the transcriptome of an organism, allowing inference of phylogenetic relationships using transcriptomic data.

The most common approach is the comparison of homologous sequences for genes using sequence alignment techniques to identify similarity. Another application of molecular phylogeny is in DNA barcoding, wherein the species of an individual organism is identified using small sections of mitochondrial DNA or chloroplast DNA.

❑❑❑

Chapter 6

Primer Designing for Polymerase Chain Reaction

Vikas Mahajan, R.K. Taggar, Dhirendra Kumar and Nishant Kumar

The most significant factor for successful PCR is the design of primers. The primer sequence determines several things such as the length of the product, its melting temperature and ultimately the yield. A poorly designed primer can result in little or no product due to non-specific amplification or primer-dimer formation, which can become competitive enough to suppress product formation. This note is provided to give rules that should be taken into consideration, when designing primers for PCR.

Primer Selection

Several variables must be taken into account when designing PCR primers. Among the most critical are:

a) Primer Length

Since both specificity and the temperature and time of annealing are at least partly dependent on primer length, this parameter is most critical for successful PCR. In general, oligonucleotides between 18 and 24 bases are extremely sequence specific, provided that the annealing temperature is optimal. Primer length is also proportional to annealing efficiency: in general, the longer the primer, more inefficient the annealing. With fewer templates primed at each step, this can result in a significant decrease in amplified product. The primers should not be too short, however, unless the application specifically calls for it. As discussed below, the goal should be to design a primer with an annealing temperature of at least 50°C.

b) Melting Temperature (T_m)

The relationship between annealing temperature and melting temperature is one of the "Black Boxes" of PCR. A general thumb rule use an annealing temperature that is 5°C lower than the melting temperature. Thus, when aiming for an annealing temperature of at least 50°C, this corresponds to a primer with a calculated melting temperature (T_m) ~55°C. Often, the annealing temperature determined in this fashion will not be optimal and empirical experiments will have to be performed to determine the optimal temperature.

It is important to keep in mind that there are two primers added to a PCR reaction. Both of the oligonucleotide primers should be designed such that they have similar melting temperatures. If primers are mismatched in terms of T_m, amplification will be less efficient or may not work at all since the primer with the higher T_m will mis-prime at lower temperatures and the primer with the lower T_m may not work at higher temperatures.

The melting temperatures of oligos are most accurately calculated using nearest neighbor thermodynamic calculations with the formula:

$$\mathbf{T_m primer = \Delta H\ [\Delta S + R\ In\ (c/4)]\ -273.15°C + 16.6\ log\ 10\ [K+]}$$

Where,

H is the enthalpy and S is the entropy for helix formation, R is the molar gas constant and c is the concentration of primer. This is most easily accomplished using any of a number of primer design software packages on the market. Fortunately, a good working approximation of this value (generally valid for oligos in the 18-24 base range) can be calculated using the formula:

$$\mathbf{T_m = 2(A+T) + 4(G+C)}$$

The table below shows calculated values for primers of various lengths using this equation, which is known as the Wallace formula, and assuming a 50% GC content. The temperatures calculated using Wallace's rule are inaccurate at the extremes of this chart.

In addition to calculating the melting temperatures of the primers, care must be taken to ensure that the melting temperature of the product is low enough to ensure 100% melting at 92°C. This parameter will help ensure a more efficient PCR, but is not always necessary for successful PCR.

Primer Length	Tm = 2 (A+T) + 4(G+C)	Primer Length	Tm = 2 (A+T) + 4(G+C)
4	12°C	22	66°C
6	18°C	24	72°C
8	24°C	26	78°C
10	30°C	28	84°C
12	36°C	30	90°C
14	42°C	32	96°C
16	48°C	34	102°C
18	54°C	36	108°C
20	60°C	38	114°C

In general, products between 100-600 base pairs are efficiently amplified in many PCR reactions. If there is doubt, the product Tm can be calculated using the formula:

$$T_m = 81.5 + 16.6 (\log 10 [K+] + 0.41 (\%G+C)-675/\text{length}$$

Under standard PCR conditions of 50 mM KCL, this reduces to

$$T_m = 59.9 + 0.41 (\%G+C) - 675/\text{length}$$

c) Specificity

As mentioned above, primer specificity is at least partly dependent on primer length. It is evident that there are many more unique 24 base oligos than there are 15 base pair oligos. That being said, primers must be chosen so that they have a unique sequence within the template DNA that is to be amplified. A primer designed with a highly repetitive sequence will result in a smear when amplifying genomic DNA. However, the same primer may give a single band if a single clone from a genomic library is amplified. Because Taq Polymerase is active over a broad range of temperatures, primer extension will occur at the lower temperatures of annealing. If the temperature is too low, non-specific priming may occur which can be extended by the polymerase if there is a short homology at the 3' end. In general, a melting temperature of 55°C -72°C gives the best results.

d) G/C Content and Polypyrimidine (T, C) or Polypurine (A, G) Stretches

The base composition of primers should be between 45-55% GC. The primer sequence must be chosen such that there is no PolyG or

PolyC stretches that can promote non-specific annealing. Poly A and Poly T stretches are also to be avoided as these will "breath" and open up stretches of the primer-template complex. This can lower the efficiency of amplification. Polypyrimidine (T, C) and polypurine (A, G) stretches should also be avoided. Ideally the primer will have a near random mix of nucleotides, a 50% GC content and be ~20 bases long. This will put the Tm in the range of 56°C - 62°C.

e) 3'-End Sequence

It is well established that the 3' terminal position in PCR primers is essential for the control of mis-priming. We have already explored the problem of primer homologies occurring at these regions. Another variable to look at is the inclusion of a G or C residue at the 3' end of primers. This "GC Clamp" helps to ensure correct binding at the 3' end due to the stronger hydrogen bonding of G/C residues. It also helps to improve the efficiency of the reaction by minimizing any "breathing" that might occur.

f) GC Clamp

The presence of G or C bases within the last five bases from the 3' end of primers (GC clamp) helps promote specific binding at the 3' end due to the stronger bonding of G and C bases. More than 3 G's or C's should be avoided in the last 5 bases at the 3' end of the primer.

g) Primer Secondary Structures

Presence of the primer secondary structures produced by intermolecular or intramolecular interactions can lead to poor or no yield of the product. They adversely affect primer template annealing and thus the amplification. They greatly reduce the availability of primers to the reaction.

i) **Hairpins:** It is formed by intramolecular interaction within the primer and should be avoided. Optimally a 3' end hairpin with a ÄG of -2 kcal/mol and an internal hairpin with a ÄG of -3 kcal/mol is tolerated generally.

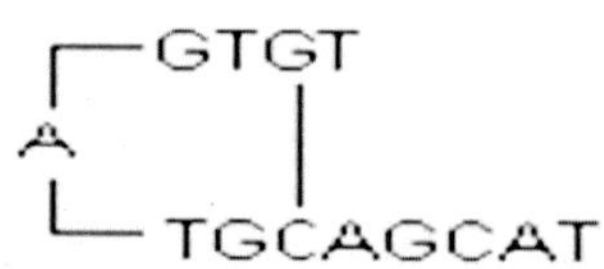

ΔG definition: The Gibbs free energy G is the measure of the amount of work that can be extracted from a process operating at a constant pressure. It is the measure of the spontaneity of the reaction. The stability of hairpin is commonly represented by its ΔG value, the energy required to break the secondary structure. Larger negative value for ΔG indicates stable, undesirable hairpins. Presence of hairpins at the 3' end most adversely affects the reaction.

$$\Delta G = \Delta H - T\Delta S$$

ii) **Self Dimer:** A primer self-dimer is formed by intermolecular interactions between the two (same sense) primers, where the primer is homologous to itself. Generally a large amount of primers are used in PCR compared to the amount of target gene. When primers form intermolecular dimers much more readily than hybridizing to target DNA, they reduce the product yield. Optimally a 3' end self dimer with a ΔG of -5 kcal/mol and an internal self dimer with a ΔG of -6 kcal/mol is tolerated generally.

iii) **Cross Dimer:** Primer cross dimers are formed by intermolecular interaction between sense and antisense primers, where they are homologous. Optimally a 3' end cross dimer with a ΔG of -5 kcal/mol and an internal cross dimer with a ΔG of -6 kcal/mol is tolerated generally.

```
         5' TGTGATGCAGCATCACGCACAC 3'
              || ||        ||
3' CTACGTCGACTCTGATAGCTACG 5'
```

h) Repeats

A repeat is a di-nucleotide occurring many times consecutively and should be avoided because they can misprime. For example: ATATATAT. A maximum number of di-nucleotide repeats acceptable in an oligo is 4 di-nucleotides.

i) Runs

Primers with long runs of a single base should generally be avoided as they can misprime. For example, AGCGGGGGATGGGG has runs of base 'G' of value 5 and 4. A maximum number of runs accepted is 4bp.

j) 3' End Stability

It is the maximum ÄG value of the five bases from the 3' end. An unstable 3' end (less negative ÄG) will result in less false priming.

k) Avoid Template Secondary Structure

A single stranded Nucleic acid sequences is highly unstable and fold into conformations (secondary structures). The stability of these template secondary structures depends largely on their free energy and melting temperatures (Tm). Consideration of template secondary structures is important in designing primers, especially in qPCR. If primers are designed on a secondary structures which is stable even above the annealing temperatures, the primers are unable to bind to the template and the yield of PCR product is significantly affected. Hence, it is important to design primers in the regions of the templates that do not form stable secondary structures during the PCR reaction. Our products determine the secondary structures of the template and design primers avoiding them.

l) Avoid Cross Homology

To improve specificity of the primers it is necessary to avoid regions of homology. Primers designed for a sequence must not amplify other genes in the mixture. Commonly, primers are designed and then BLASTed to test the specificity. Our products offer a better alternative. You can avoid regions of cross homology while designing primers. You can BLAST the templates against the appropriate non-redundant database and the software will interpret the results. It will identify regions significant cross homologies in each template and avoid them during primer search.

Parameters for Primer Pair Design

1. **Amplicon Length**

   The amplicon length is dictated by the experimental goals. For qPCR, the target length is closer to 100 bp and for standard PCR, it is near 500 bp. If you know the positions of each primer with respect to the template, the product is calculated as:

   Product length = (Position of antisense primer-Position of sense primer) + 1.

2. **Product Position**

   Primer can be located near the 5' end, the 3' end or anywhere within specified length. Generally, the sequence close to the 3' end is known with greater confidence and hence preferred most frequently.

3. **Tm of Product**

   Melting Temperature (Tm) is the temperature at which one half of the DNA duplex will dissociate and become single stranded. The stability of the primer-template DNA duplex can be measured by the melting temperature (Tm).

4. **Optimum Annealing Temperature (Ta Opt)**

   The formula of Rychlik is most respected. Our products use this formula to calculate it and thousands of our customers have reported good results using it for the annealing step of the PCR cycle. It usually results in good PCR product yield with minimum false product production.

   Ta Opt = 0.3 (Tm of primer) + 0.7 (Tm of product) - 14.9

   Where,

   Tm of primer is the melting temperature of the less stable primer-template pair

   Tm of product is the melting temperature of the PCR product.

5. **Primer Pair Tm Mismatch Calculation**

   The two primers of a primer pair should have closely matched melting temperatures for maximizing PCR product yield. The difference of 5°C or more can lead no amplification.

Conclusion

It is essential that care is taken in the design of primers for PCR. Several parameters including the length of the primer, %GC content and the 3' sequence need to be optimized for successful PCR. Certain of these parameters can be easily manually optimized while others are best done with commercial computer programs. In any event, careful observance of the general rules of primer design will help ensure successful experiments.

❑❑❑

Chapter 7

Analysis of Orthologous and Paralogous Genes in Animal Genomes

Sachinandan De and Biswajit Brahma

Analysis the evolution of gene families, the phylogeny of species, and tracing the biogeography of populations depend on reliable delineation of orthologous genes and paralogous copies of them. Orthologous genes are the genes that are originated from a single gene in the last common ancestor of the compared species. Each of the delineated orthologous groups (OGs) can also include species- or lineage-specific gene copies (inparalogs), that evolved by gene duplication after the evolutionary split of the ancestor into different species. Finally, horizontal gene transfer can give rise to xenologous gene copies (xenologs) from a single ancestral gene. Orthologs have been used not only as evolutionary markers to infer species phylogenies but also to link functionally equivalent genes across genomes, thus allowing annotation of unknown proteins in other species (Brief Bioinformatics. 2011; 12: 379–91).

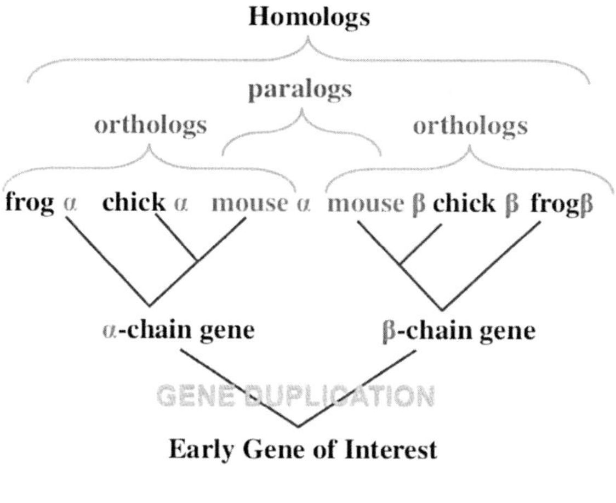

Two fundamentally different approaches to identify potential orthologs, paralogs, and xenologs have been established: tree-based and graph-based approaches. The benefit of graph-based approaches, which we will subsequently focus on, is their computational efficiency and scalability (Brief Bioinformatics. 2011;12:379–91.). No single prediction method holds a clear advantage over the other, and their usage is typically dependent on the requirements of the problem that must be addressed, systematic descriptions and comparisons of these methods including advantages and pitfalls can be found in. Phylogenetic or tree-based methods that cluster genes and aim for the reconciliation of the protein and the species trees. In general, graph-based approaches (also known as pairwise sequence alignment) assessing gene orthology make use of the genome-wide best reciprocal hit (BRH) criterion. It rests on the assumption that orthologs in two genomes are more similar to each other than to any other gene in the compared genomes, since they are direct and exclusive descendants from a single ancestral gene (PLoS Comput Biol. 2012;8(5): 1002514.). Graph-based methods include 2 steps: first, pairs of ortholog genes are detected, and graphs, with nodes representing genes and edges representing relationships, are defined; second, clusters of ortholog genes are organized based on the structure of the graphs. The simplest approaches identify orthologs between genes in pair of genomes(Methods Mol Biol. 2012; 855:259-79).The key assumption is that orthologs are those genes among homologs with the minimum divergence. Orthologs from 2 genomes are all those genes detected as being the reciprocal best hit of each other (Proc Natl Acad Sci U S A. 2005, 102(25):8791-2). This widespread methodology is generally defined as the search for the Bidirectional Best Hit (BBH).The BBH detection between 2 genomes is computationally efficient because sequence alignments can be computed by well-established approaches, either based on dynamic programming (J Mol Biol. 1981 Mar 25; 147:195-7)or on more efficient heuristic algorithms, such as the BLAST set of programs (Bioinformatics. 2008; 24:319-24). The BBH detection has some constraints. Some genes in a species can have more than 1 ortholog with another species. This can reflect a gene duplication after a speciation event, whereas the ortholog counterpart in the other genome remains in single copy, namely, a singleton gene.

The phylogenetic methods tend to be robust and accurate, they do not scale well (computationally) with the number of input sequences and are sensitive to the strategies applied in each of the four steps. To alleviate some of the challenges associated to phylogeny-based orthology prediction, particularly the computational scalability with number of input sequences, pairwise sequence alignment methods were developed.

Sequence similarity is a strong indication of orthology among genes or proteins, these methods are typically performed using a reciprocal best BLAST hit (RBBH) approach. While RBBH detection is computationally fast, it has its own drawbacks, such as being affected by incomplete genome sequences or gene loss, therefore incorrectly predicting a paralog as an ortholog. Nevertheless, in particular circumstances where trusted orthologs are required, such as information enrichment in genome annotation

Protein sequences have been the widespread exploited reference to identify orthology relationships, mainly because these analyses are useful to find functional counterparts among species. However, orthology should refer to evolutionary relationships traceable at genome level. Similarity at protein sequence level does not always represent similarity at gene level. Indeed, it does not permit to exploit similarities embedded in untranslated regions (UTRs), or may lead to misinterpretations due to open reading frame (ORF) mis assignments, difficult to be detected because of the lack of consistent confirmatory data at proteome level, or to sequencing errors.

Gene orthology detection software tools

UCSC Genome Browser

Offers online public access to a growing database of genomic sequence and annotations for a large collection of organisms, primarily vertebrates, with an emphasis on the human and mouse genomes. The Browser's web-based tools provide an integrated environment for visualizing, comparing, analysing and sharing both publicly available and user-generated genomic data sets. The browser has data sets available on the most recent human assembly, hg38/GRCh38, to include updated gene prediction sets from GENCODE, more phenotype- and disease-associated variants from ClinVar and ClinGen, more genomic regulatory data, and a new multiple genome alignment.

ParameciumDB

Provides data about the model organism *Paramecium tetraurelia*. ParameciumDB was created by using components of the Generic Model Organism Database (GMOD). It offers data about gene expression data from genome-wide transcriptome experiments using a NimbleGen custom microarray platform. The database can be consulted through a detailed view that provides protein alignments and links to external databases.

BLASTP

The Basic Local Alignment Search Tool (BLAST) (Altschul *et al.*, 1990, 1997) is probably the most common heuristic algorithm used to find homologs. During the database phase, BLAST decomposes the query into small *words* and compares them to words in the database to find the most promising target sequences for alignment (Altschul *et al.*, 1990). The final scores produced by BLAST might mainly be affected by two options: Masking of low-information segments and the method to produce the final alignments. Low information segments of sequence are commonly masked (marked to be ignored), because these segments might initiate too many spurious alignments of a query with unrelated targets.

OMA

The OMA ("Orthologous MAtrix") project is a method and database for the inference of orthologs among complete genomes. The distinctive features of OMA are its broad scope and size, high quality of inferences, feature-rich web interface, availability of data in a wide range of formats and interfaces, and frequent update schedule of two releases per year.

OMA's inference algorithm consists of three main phases. First, to infer homologous sequences (sequences of common ancestry), all-against-all Smith-Waterman alignments are computed and significant matches are retained. Second, to infer orthologous pairs (the subset of homologs related by speciation events), mutually closest homologs are identified based on evolutionary distances, taking into account distance inference uncertainty and the possibility for differential gene losses. Third, these orthologs are clustered to identify cliques of orthologous pairs ("OMA groups"), which are useful as marker genes for phylogenetic reconstruction and tend to be very specific; and to identify hierarchical orthologous groups ("HOGs"), groups of genes defined for particular taxonomic ranges and identify all genes that have descended from a common ancestral gene in that taxonomic range. The OMA pipeline can also run on custom genomic/ transcriptomic data using the OMA stand-alone software, and it is even possible to combine precomputed data with custom data by exporting parts of the OMA database.

orthAgogue

A tool for high speed estimation of homology relations within and between species in massive data sets. orthAgogue is one of the popular heuristic approaches and comprises three major steps: a) Performing an all-against-all BLAST b) Identification of putative orthology and inparalogy relations with the Inparanoid algorithm c)Generation of disjoint clusters of closely related proteins with the Markov Clustering Algorithm (MCL).

primeGEM

Computes for a pair of genes the probability that they are orthologous. primeGEM is a program that performs probabilistic orthology analysis. This framework is based on the gene evolution model. primeGEM is a program that performs probabilistic orthology analysis (Arvestad et al. 2003, 2004, submitted, Sennblad and Lagergren, 2009). It computes for a pair of genes the probability that they are orthologous (note that this corresponds to the probability that their least common ancestor is a speciation). It is based on the *gene evolution model* which models gene duplication and loss.

OrthoReD

OrthoReD (**Ortho**logy predictions from **Re**duced **D**atasets) represents a tree-building-based orthology prediction tool designed to be executed on desktop computers with accuracy comparable to other published tree-building-based tools. The computational requirement is minimized by 1) generating a reduced dataset only for each gene of interest, and 2) limiting the number of genes that enter the tree-building step.

DLRSOrthology

DLRSOrthology is a program for probabilistic orthology analysis using an integrated gene evolution and sequence evolution models. It is based on DLRS (pronounced *Delirius* and previously known as primeGSR). DLRS is an acronym for Duplication, Loss, Rate and Sequence evolution.

WORMHOLE

WORMHOLE is a novel ortholog prediction meta-tool that applies machine learning to integrate 17 distinct ortholog prediction algorithms to identify novel least diverged orthologs (LDOs) between 6 eukaryotic species—humans, mice, zebrafish, fruit flies, nematodes, and budding yeast. Machine learning allows WORMHOLE to intelligently incorporate predictions from a wide-spectrum of strategies in order to form aggregate predictions of LDOs with high confidence. WORMHOLE is particularly adept at improving LDO prediction performance between distantly related species, expanding the pool of LDOs while maintaining low evolutionary distance and a high level of functional relatedness between genes in LDO pairs.

ORCAN

ORCAN (ORtholog sCANner) is a web-based meta-server for one-click evolutionary and functional annotation of protein sequences. The server combines information from the most popular orthology-prediction resources, including four tools and four online databases. Functional annotation utilizes five additional comparisons between the query and identified homologs, including: sequence similarity, protein domain architectures, functional motifs, Gene Ontology term assignments and a list of associated articles. Furthermore, the server uses a plurality-based rating system to evaluate the orthology relationships and to rank the reference proteins by their evolutionary and functional relevance to the query.

OGCleaner

Orthology Group Cleaner (the OGCleaner), a tool designed for filtering putative orthology groups as homology or non-homology clusters by considering all sequences in a cluster. Filters putative homology clusters of amino acid sequences by using machine learning algorithms based on annotated orthology clusters. The OGCleaner relies on high-quality orthologous groups identified in OrthoDB to train machine learning algorithms that are able to distinguish between true-positive and false-positive homology groups. This package aims to improve the quality of phylogenetic tree construction especially in instances of lower-quality transcriptome assemblies.

DeNoGAP

De-novo genome analysis pipeline (DeNoGAP) is an automated, iterative and high-throughput analysis of data from comparative genomics projects involving hundreds of whole genome sequences. The pipeline is able to perform reference-assisted and de novo gene prediction, homolog protein family assignment, ortholog prediction, functional annotation, and pan-genome analysis using a range of proven tools and databases. DeNoGAP scales linearly since the homology assignment is based on iteratively refined hidden Markov models. This iterative clustering strategy enables DeNoGAP to handle a very large number of genomes using minimal computational resources. Moreover, the modular structure of the pipeline permits easy updates as new analysis programs become available.

HaMStR

HaMStR is a tool to mine EST data for the presence of orthologs to a curated set of genes. HaMStR combines a profile Hidden Markov Model search and a subsequent BLAST search to extend existing ortholog cluster with sequences from further taxa. HaMStR exhibits a very low false positive rate (FDR) and good sensitivity.

OrthoFinder

OrthoFinder, a novel method that infers orthogroups of protein coding genes. It is fast, easy to use and scalable to thousands of genomes. OrthoFinder use phylogenetic methods to validate the orthogroups. Algorithm can be found at *www.stevekellylab.com/software/orthofinder* and a standalone implementation of the algorithm is available under the GPLv3 licence at *https://github.com/davidemms/OrthoFinder*.

OrthoVenn

OrthoVenn is a web platform for comparison and annotation of orthologous gene clusters among multiple species. No installation or registration is required. It works on any operating system with a modern browser and Javascript enabled. OrthoVenn provides comprehensive coverage of vertebrates, metazoa, protists, fungi, plants and bacteria for identify orthologous gene clusters and supports user define species to upload customized protein sequences. OrthoVenn has an efficient and interactive graphic tool which provide a Venn diagram view for comparing two to six species protein sequences. The only thing user need to do is choosing species or upload protein sequences.

OrthoMaM

The EnsEMBL database has been used to determine a set of orthologous genes from 12 available complete mammalian genomes. As targets for possible amplification and sequencing in additional taxa, more than 3,000 exons of length > 400 bp have been selected, among which 118, 368, 608, and 674 are respectively retrieved for 12, 11, 10, and 9 species. A bioinformatic pipeline has been developed to provide evolutionary descriptors for these candidate markers in order to assess their potential phylogenetic utility. The resulting OrthoMaM (Orthologous Mammalian Markers) database can be queried and alignments can be downloaded through a dedicated web interface http://kimura.univ-montp2.fr/orthomam.

OrthoClust

OrthoClust, a novel network-based framework for clustering data across multiple species. OrthoClust integrates the networks of individual species using orthology relationships of genes between species. As connected genes within a species and orthologous pairs across species connect genes with the same function within and across species, respectively, OrthoClust naturally extends the idea of functional modules into a cross-species dimension. The essence of OrthoClust is a cost function for the detection of modules across species.

EvoCor

Predicts genes involved in affecting specific cellular processes together with a gene of interest. EvoCor detects functional relationships among genes through *evo*lutionary analysis and gene expression *cor*relation. This web server integrates profiles of sequence divergence derived by a Hidden Markov Model (HMM) and tissue-wide gene expression patterns to determine putative functional linkages between pairs of genes. This server is easy to use and freely available at http://pilot-hmm.vbi.vt.edu/.

RecBlast

RecBlast is an intuitive and easy-to-use pipeline that enables fast and easy discovery of orthologues along and across the evolutionary tree. RecBlast is capable of running heavy, large-scale and complex Reciprocal Blast comparisons across multiple genes and multiple taxa, in a completely automatic way. RecBlast is available as a cloud-based web server, which includes an easy-to-use user interface, implemented using cloud computing and an elastic and scalable server architecture. RecBlast is also available as a powerful standalone software supporting multi-processing for large datasets, and a cloud image which can be easily deployed on Amazon Web Services cloud.

HOMECAT

HOMECAT (HOmology Mapper for Enrichment and Comparative Analysis with Translation) is a Cytoscape plugin allowing cross-species data comparison with a particular emphasis on functional genomic data (i.e. microarrays and other high throughput biological data sources). The aim at the basis of this software is to ease knowledge transfer from different species. Networks can be enriched with orthologs from other species, in the desired format.

Orthology assessment is a complex task, user can combine different sources of homology prediction, with different specificity and sensitivity, to allow achieving the desired level of precision and coverage.

The data integration is eased by the possibility of choosing between nearly 30 identifiers formats (Uniprot, RefSeq, Ensembl, etc.) and 71 microarrays platforms identifiers (including Affymetrix, Illumina and Agilent) designed for the 30 organisms supported by the current version. Homology data can be used to enrich existing networks or to create new data visualization that improve external data loading and mapping. A specific interface allows the download of curated data directly from Array Express ATLAS database, and several functionalities ease the comparison of data from different networks. Once data is integrated in the user networks any Cytoscape functionality can be used to analyze, visualize and process the data.

BUSCO

BUSCO (Benchmarking Universal Single-Copy Orthologs) provides quantitative measures for the assessment of genome assembly, gene set, and transcriptome completeness, based on evolutionarily-informed expectations of gene content from near-universal single-copy orthologs selected from OrthoDB. BUSCO assessments are implemented in open-source software, with a large selection of lineage-specific sets of Benchmarking Universal Single-Copy Orthologs. These conserved orthologs are ideal candidates for large-scale phylogenomics studies, and the annotated BUSCO gene models built during genome assessments provide a comprehensive gene predictor training set for use as part of genome annotation pipelines.

Hieranoid: hierarchical orthology inference.

Hieranoid is an orthology inference method using a hierarchical approach. Hieranoid performs pairwise orthology analysis using InParanoid at each node in a guide tree as it progresses from its leaves to the root. This concept reduces the total runtime complexity from a quadratic to a linear function of the number of species. The tree hierarchy provides a natural structure in multi-species ortholog groups, and the aggregation of multiple sequences allows for multiple alignment similarity searching techniques, which can yield more accurate ortholog groups.

'Fast Approximate Tree Classification' (FAT-CAT)

The PhyloFacts 'Fast Approximate Tree Classification' (FAT-CAT) web server provides a novel approach to ortholog identification using subtree hidden Markov model-based placement of protein sequences to phylogenomic orthology groups in the PhyloFacts database. Results on a data set of microbial, plant and animal proteins demonstrate FAT-CAT's high precision at separating orthologs and paralogs and robustness to promiscuous domains. We also present results documenting the precision of ortholog identification based on subtree hidden Markov model scoring. The FAT-CAT phylogenetic placement is used to derive a functional annotation for the query, including confidence scores and drill-down capabilities.

MultiMSOAR

An extension of MSOAR 2.0 to multiple genomes, MultiMSOAR presents a new combinatorial approach for constructing ortholog groups. MultiMSOAR allows gene losses within an ortholog group and ortholog groups involving genes only from a subset of the genomes. It also attempts to minimize the number of gene births, losses and duplications within a gene family when assigning ortholog groups. Moreover, compared with many other ortholog assignment tools for multiple genomes, MultiMSOAR 2.0 can provide more information about genome evolution in terms of gene births, losses as well as duplications.

□□□

Chapter 8

Drug Designing: Basic Concept and *in silico* Essential Tools

Akhilesh Upgade and Vikas Mahajan

Drug designing

DRUG is neither a noun nor a grammatical synonym limited to a language, rather its a designation given to a a substance after a judging its ability in diagnosis, cure, relief, treatment or prevention of disease, or intended to affect the structure or function of the body. It is a legal definition of the drug. The development of any potential drug begins with years of scientific study to determine the biochemistry behind a disease, for which pharmaceutical intervention is possible. Drug discovery was and is a time and cost consuming since a decade. Hence to ease the process computational methods are now being used. The objective of drug design is to find a chemical compound that can fit to a specific cavity on a protein target both geometrically and chemically.

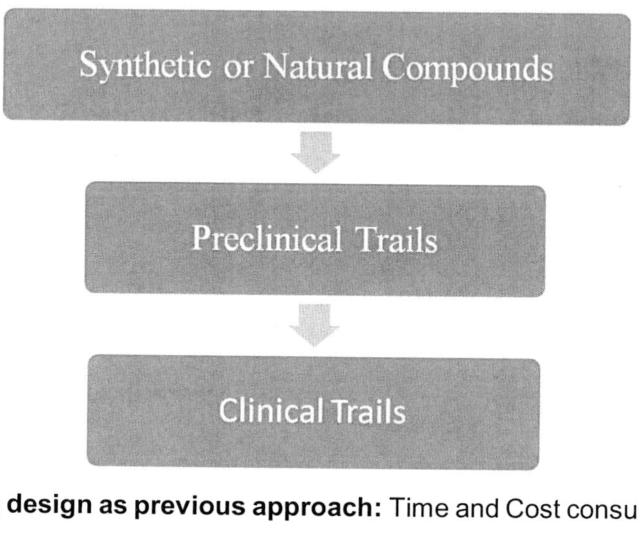

Drug design as previous approach: Time and Cost consuming

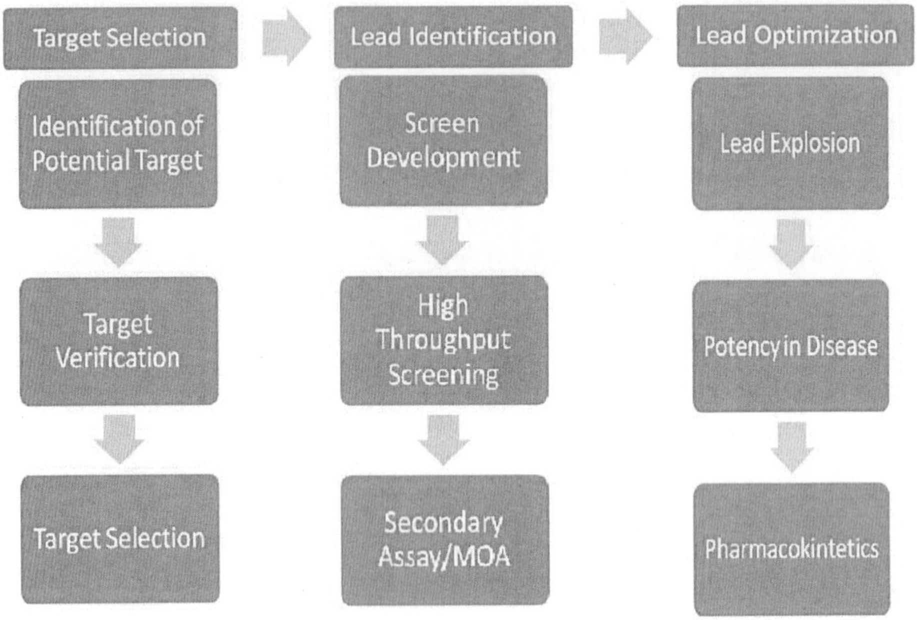

Modern drug designing approach (CADD)

Types of drug design

(1) Ligand based drug design, (2) Structure based drug design.

1. **Ligand based drug design** : Ligand-based drug design relies on knowledge of other molecules that bind to the biological target of interest used to derive a pharmacophore, homology modelling, NMR spectroscopy, x-ray crystallography, Structure based drug design.

2. **Structure-based drug design** relies on knowledge of the three dimensional structure of the biological target obtained through methods such as automated computational procedures for the intuition of a medicinal chemist & interactive graphics. This is considered as one of the most innovative and powerful approaches in drug design. SBDD is an iterative approach. It requires three-dimensional (3D) structure of the target protein, preferentially complexed with a ligand, where binding mode, affinity and confirmation of a ligand binding can be discerned.

CADD represents computational methods and resources that are used to facilitate the design and discovery of new therapeutic solutions.

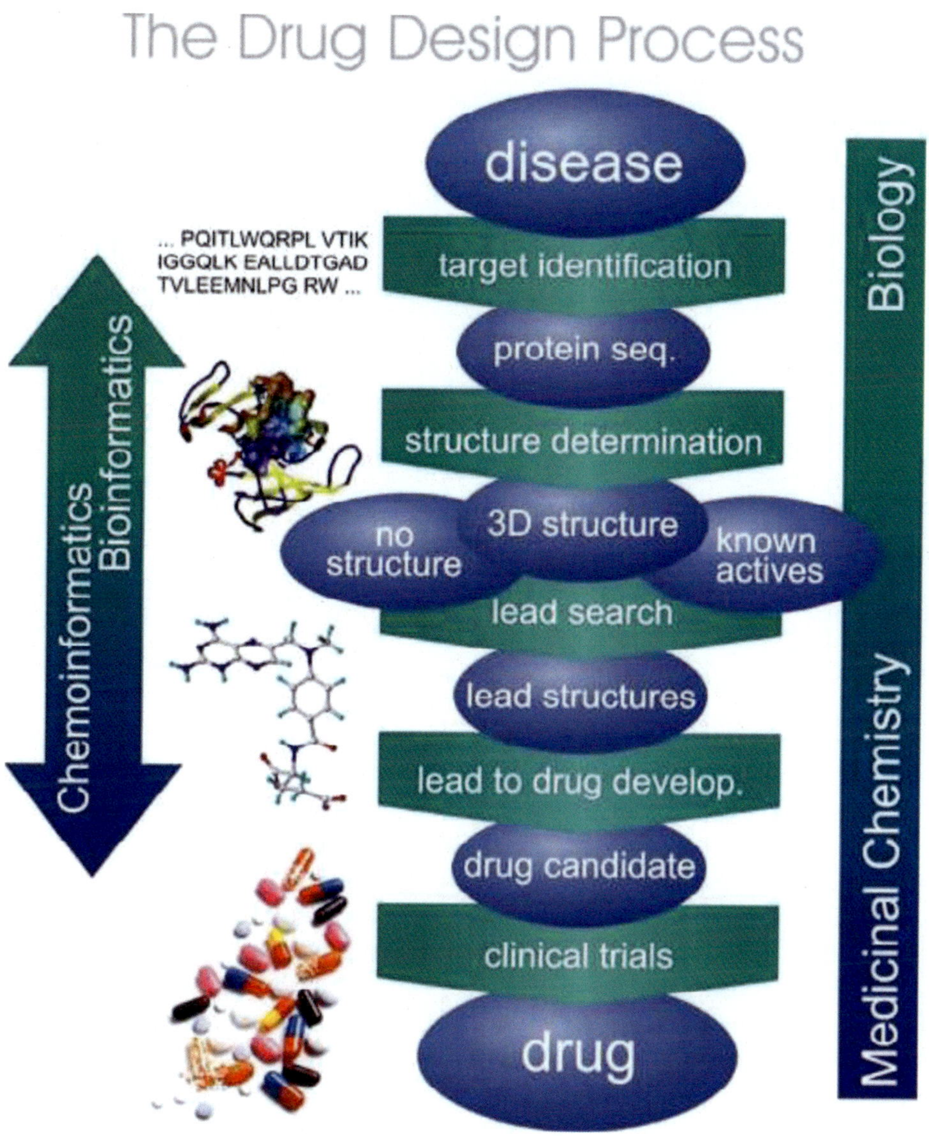

General pathway for CADD

Mechanism based drug design

When the disease process is understood at the molecular level and the target molecule(s) are defined, drugs can be designed specifically to interact with the target molecule in such a way as to disrupt the disease.

Selection of disease

The first step in the design of drugs to treat diseases is to determine the biochemical basis of the disease process. Ideally, one would know the various steps involved in the physiological pathway that carries out the normal function. In addition, one would know the exact step(s) in the pathway that are altered in the diseased state. Knowledge about the regulation of the pathway is also important. Finally, one would know the three- dimensional structures of the molecules involved in the process

Target selection

There are potentially many ways in which biochemical pathways could become abnormal and result in disease. Therefore, knowledge of the molecular basis of the disease is important in order to select a target at which to disrupt the process. Categories of targets: enzymes, receptors, nucleic acids.

Structure Determination

Desired protein or the receptor can be taken from the various databases most important database and reliable is Protein data bank (PDB). It act as a biological resource of macromolecules. Every enzyme or receptor has their own designated id given by PDB and by this anyone can access the same. X ray crystallographic data of the protein or NMR based structures are generally available in the database which can be download and it also shows internally binded small molecules and docked compounds or inhibitors like metal ions. The Universal Protein Resource (UniProt) is a comprehensive resource for protein sequence and annotation data. The UniProt databases are the uniprot Knowledgebase (UniProtKB), the UniProt Reference Clusters (UniRef), and the uniprot Archive (uniParc). uniprot is a collaboration between the European Bioinformatics Institute (EMBL-EBI), the SIB Swiss Institute of Bioinformatics and the Protein Information Resource (PIR). Every structure can be retrieved in 3D format known as 'pdb' e.g. 4H0D.pdb. Visualization of the Proteiin structure in 3D needs visualizer like Accelrys Discovery Studio, RasMol, J Mol or Chimera open licence software.

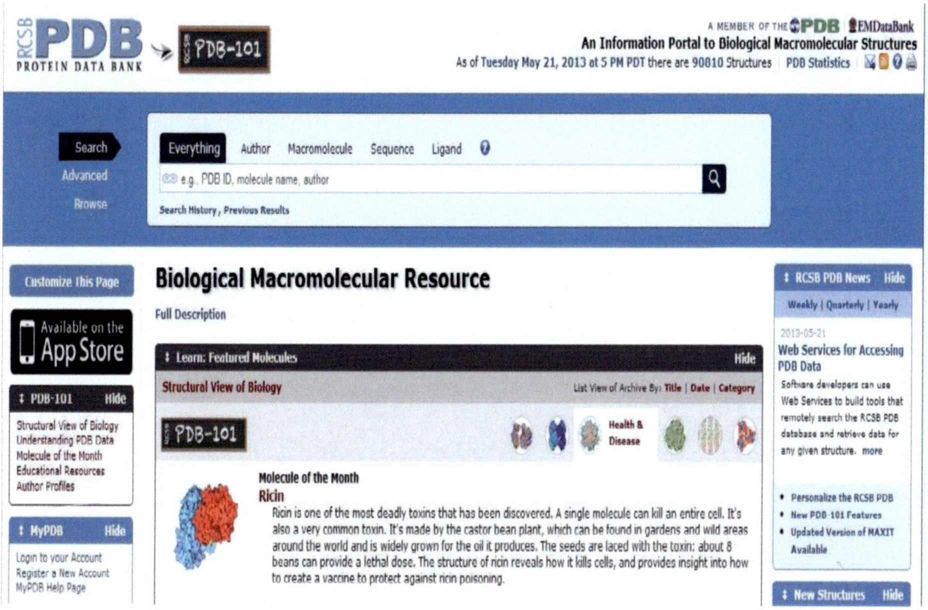

Determination of Actives Site

Various platforms are available for this which gives Ramachandran plot of the protein to understand allowed region in which we are going to select target site. E.g. Pro Pred, Promate. Pocket finder Its nothing but a chain of amino acid which forms a cleft/ pocket and that can be active site. We need to define active site before drug targeting, Now a days set of softwares available in which it automatically identifies sites and get attached.

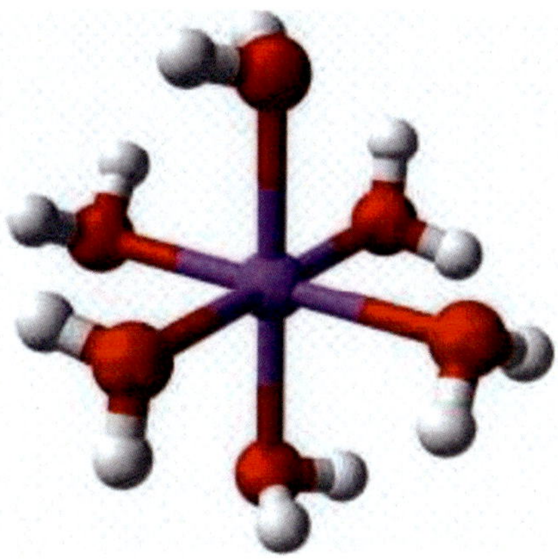

Selection of the small molecule/ Ligand

Basic requirement of Computer

- Operating system: Windows 7 enterprise 32 bit operating system
- Processor: Intel[R], Core[TM]i3-3220 CPU @ 3.30GHz
- Installed memory [RAM]: minimum 2GB
- Hard disk: 500 GB
- Graphic cards NVIDEA

Internet facilities and Softwares

1. **Discovery studio**

   Discovery Studio is a suite of software for simulating small molecule and macromolecule systems. It is developed and distributed by Accelrys. The product suite has a strong academic collaboration programme, supporting scientific research and makes use of a number of software algorithms developed originally in the scientific community, including CHARMM, MODELLER, DELPHI, ZDOCK, DMol3 and more.

2. **Auto dock**

   Autodock is molecular modeling simulation software. It is especially effective for protein-ligand docking. Autodock 4 is available under the GNU General Public License. Autodock Vina is available under the Apache license.

3. **Molsoft**

   Molsoft offers software tools and services in lead discovery, modeling, cheminformatics, bioinformatics, and corporate data management, and forms partnerships with biotechnology and pharmaceutical companies. Molsoft is building unique technologies for structure prediction that improves our understanding of the spatial organization of biological molecules and their interactions with each other, their biological substrates and drug-like molecules at the atomic level.

4. **UCSF chimera**

   UCSF Chimera is a highly extensible program for interactive visualization and analysis of molecular structures and related data, including density maps, supramolecular assemblies, sequence alignments, docking results, trajectories, and conformational ensembles. High-quality images and animations can be generated. Chimera includes complete documentation and several tutorials, and can be downloaded free of charge for academic, government, nonprofits, and personal use. Chimera is developed by the Resource for Bio computing, Visualization, and Informatics, funded by the National Institutes of Health.

5. **Open Babel**

   Open Babelis a chemical toolbox designed to speak the many languages of chemical data. It's an open, collaborative project allowing anyone to search, convert, analyze, or store data from molecular modelling, chemistry, solid-state materials, biochemistry, or related areas

Databases

1. **Zinc database**

   Zincis free database of commercially-available compounds for virtual screening. Zinc contains over 14 million purchasable compounds in ready-to-dock, 3D formats. Zinc is provided by the Shoichet Laboratory in the Department of Pharmaceutical Chemistry at the University of California, San Francisco (UCSF).

2. **Pubchem**

   Pubchem is a database of chemical molecules and their activities against biological assays. The system is maintained by the National Center for Biotechnology Information (NCBI), a component of the National Library of Medicine, which is part of the United States National Institutes of Health (NIH). Pubchem can be accessed for free through a web user interface. Millions of compound structures and descriptive datasets can be freely downloaded via FTP. Pubchem contains substance descriptions and small molecules with fewer than 1000 atoms and 1000 bonds. More than 80 database vendors contribute to the growing Pubchem database.

Protein characterization tools

1. **SOPM**

   Secondary structure predictionis a set of techniques in bioinformatics that aim to predict the secondary structures of proteins and nucleic acid sequences based only on knowledge of their primary structure. For proteins, this means predicting the formation of protein structures such as alpha helices and beta strands, while for nucleic acids it means predicting the formation of nucleic acid structures like helixes and stem-loop structures through base pairing and base stacking interactions.

2. **SOSUI**

   Sosuiis a free online tool that predicts a part of the secondary structure of proteins from a given amino acid sequence (AAS). The main objective is to determine whether the protein in question is a soluble or a transmembrane protein.

3. **Disulfind Tool**

   Disulfindis a server for predicting the disulfide bonding state of cysteines and their disulfide connectivity given a protein sequence.

Computational biology is vast and reliable method of drug discovery process. Consider any target downloaded from database Protein Data Bank (PDB). (PDB: http://www.rcsb.org/ pdb/home/ home.do) All water molecules need to remove and on final stage add hydrogen atoms.

Visualization of target

Discovery studio visualize

Discovery Studio visualize allows you to view and edit molecular structures, sequences and sequence alignments and Perl scripts created with the Discovery Studio and other applications. It provides a convenient interface for everyday data analysis tasks and enables you to share and view data with other collaborators.

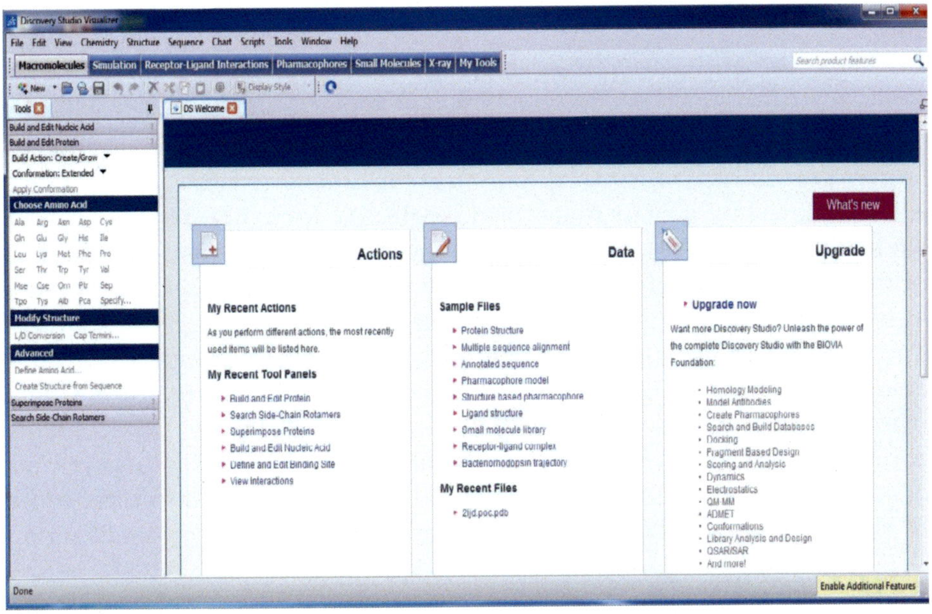

Discovery studio visualizer home page.

- Steps of target visualization
- Go to file in menu bar.
- Open PDB file of target.

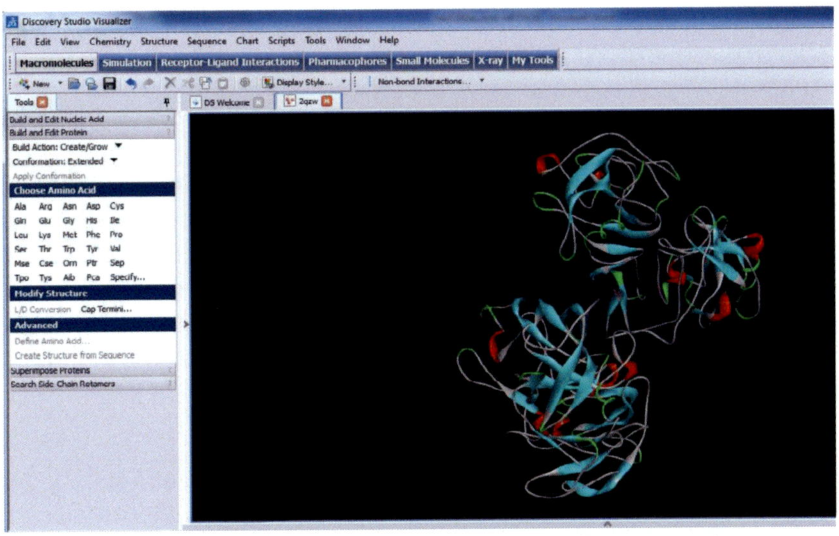

Target protein visualize in discovery studio visualizer.

Characterization of target

Proteins differ from each other in their size, molecular structure and physiochemical properties. These differences allow for protein analysis and characterization by separation and identification. Separation is typically done via electrophoresis where proteins are differentiated by size or mass, and isoelectric focusing, where protein are separated by charge. These techniques can be done independently, or in combination- referred to as 2D electrophoresis.Mass spectrometry equipment includes protein fractionators, GC/MS, LC/MS, CE/MS and time of flight systems. Identification can also be done via amino acid sequencing by Edman degradation, crystal imaging and surface plasmon resonance. With so many options available, laboratories typically will employ multiple strategies for protein analysis and characterization. Here one can characterize protein via online tools of protein characterization. Following are characterizing parameters.

- Expasy prot param tool
- SOPMA
- SOSUI
- HMMTOP
- CYS REC
- Disulfide

Ligand and chemical database

A chemical library or compound library is a collection of stored chemicals usually used ultimately in high-throughput screening or industrial manufacture. A chemical database is a database specifically designed to store chemical information. This information is about chemical and crystal structures, spectra, reactions and syntheses, and thermophysical data. A ligand is an ion or molecule that binds to a central metal atom to form a complex (alternatively known as a coordination entity). Ligands are atoms or molecules with electron pairs available; they may be neutral or negatively charged.

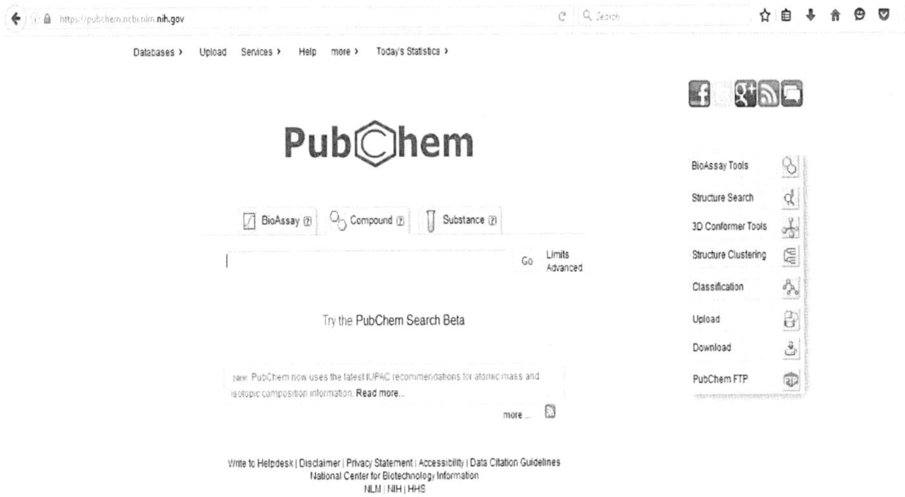

(1) PubChem
Pubchem database home page.

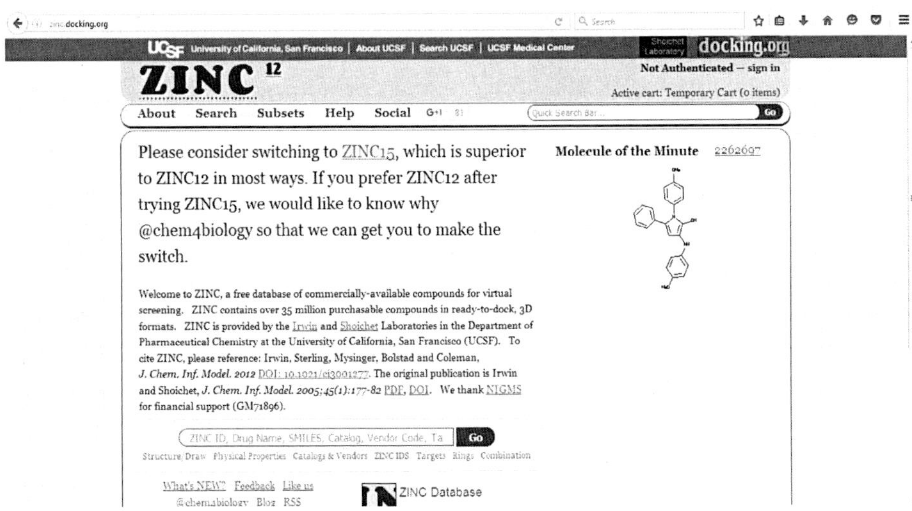

(2) ZINC database
Zinc database home page.

Molecular docking studies

Molecular docking is a key tool in structural molecular biology and computer-assisted drug design. The goal of ligand-protein docking is to predict the predominant binding mode(s) of a ligand with a protein of known three-dimensional structure.

Types of docking

- Protien- Ligand Studies
- Flexible Ligand, Rigid Receptor
- Search much Larger Space
- Search the conformational Space using Molecular Dynamic
- Protien- Protien Docking
- Both Molecule Usually Considered Rigid
- 6 Degree of freedom

Molecular docking can be done by various softwares but the alogorithm developed for each is different and gives slight variation again here is issue of validation. Currently most important and reliable tools are Accelrys Discovery Studio and Schrodinger suite followed by Autodock as a freeware. For beginner AUTODOCK is recommended.

Autodock is a suite of automated docking tools. It is designed to predict how small molecules, such as substrates or drug candidates, bind to a receptor of known 3D structure. Current distributions of autodock consist of two generations of software: autodock 4 and autodock vina. Autodock 4 actually consists of two main programs: (1) autodock performs the docking of the ligand to a set of grids describing the target protein; (2) autogrid pre-calculates these grids. In addition to using them for docking, the atomic affinity grids can be visualised. This can help, for example, to guide organic synthetic chemists design better binders. Autodock Vina does not require choosing atom types and pre-calculating grid maps for them. Instead, it calculates the grids internally, for the atom types that are needed, and it does this virtually instantly.

Interpretation of Results

Once the docking process over by the software the following data need to be tabulated which clearly shows that interaction of the molecule and compound. It is clear that entropic contribution of bond stretches and angle bends are negligible and the interaction can be seen in between amino acid and the drug compound The assumption is often done for rotational and translational entropy, although they are known to vary not only from one complex to another, but also among alternative bound conformations of a single complex.

The loss of flexibility of the ligand upon binding, resulting from a reduction of the energetically accessible rotamer has an average impact on the binding free energy ranging between -4 and -5 kcal/mol. An ideal scoring function should account for this reduction of the accessible conformational space, but this penalty is usually calculated as a function of the number of frozen dihedral angles. Hence as per current standard negative free binding energy shows better docking and score from -4.0 kcal/mol onwards considers good score. Docked compounds at specific target can be visualised any time and seen as follows.

Docked View 3D	2D Ligand plot	Hydrogen bond plot	Docking score Kcal/mol
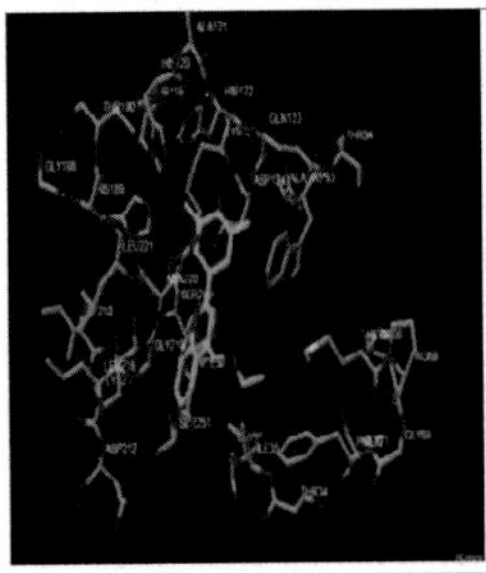	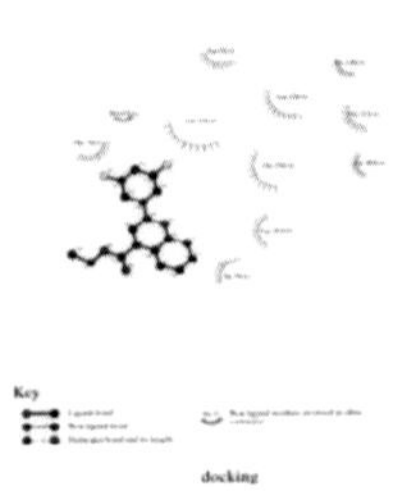	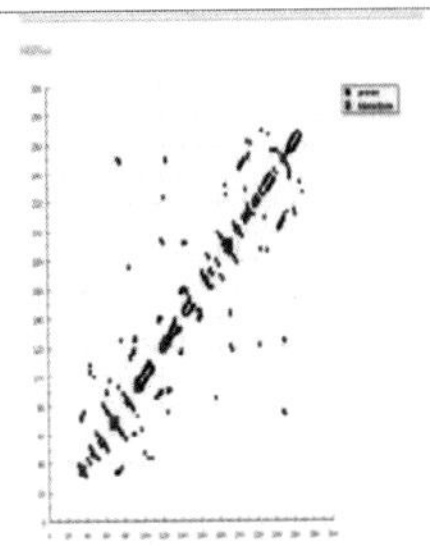	**-6.79 kcal/mol**

Way of presenting the data when a confirmation of the ligand and receptor is binded with perfect poses. Every ligand takes best pose unless it is not stable and fixes a bond with interacting amino acid of the target which result into release of energy.

Binding the drug into designated pocket of the target doesn t mean that the drug is designed it still required to analyse the compound whether the drug is really capable of by using tool ADMET.

ADME is an abbreviation in pharmacokinetics and pharmacology for "absorption, distribution, metabolism, and excretion," and describes the disposition of a pharmaceuticalcompound within an organism. The four criteria all influence the drug levels and kinetics of drug exposure to the tissues and hence influence the performance and pharmacological activity of the compound as a drug.

❑ Absorption

As word itself is self explanatory, Absorption refers to a processes that a drug entering into the blood (The reason why a drug must pass into the bloodstream, is that it aims to reach its target tissue in the body, unless there is a direct injection to the site of action).

Typically, before it can reach the target cells, a drug has to get through surfaces such as the digestive tract. However, absorption can be affected by many factors, such as blood flow, pain stress, intestinal transit time, chemical instability in the stomach, poor compound solubility, and inability to permeate the intestinal wall, etc. All of these can reduce the absorption effect of medicine when it is taken.

❒ Distribution

When we talk about the absorption, we actually know about distribution. Usually, before a dug is being absorbed, it has to be transported to tissues and organs via the blood stream. Distribution is kind like how a drug moving throughout the body, and it is regarded as the drug transfer between one tissue or organ to another. However, the drug distribution can also be affected by some factors, such as blood flow rates, polarity and binding to serum proteins, or molecular size, etc. Besides, when a drug meets some natural barriers like the blood!! brain barrier, the distribution can be a serious problem.

❒ Metabolism

Usually, a drug begins to be metabolized since it enters the body. This is because our bodies recognize those drugs and chemicals as foreign substances, and thus metabolism has to be proceed so that it can make these "foreign substances" more hydrophilic and successfully reach the next level Excretion, otherwise those drugs and chemicals will be reabsorbed and remain in the body for prolonged periods.

❒ Excretion

After distribution and metabolism, here comes the next level Excretion. It means the "foreign substances" can finally get out of our bodies, which frequently occurs in the urine and feces, or through the lungs as gases. In addition, excretion can also be realized by some natural routes, such as tears, sweat, breath and saliva. For patients who have kidney or liver problems, they have to be more cautious and careful about the medicine they take, because they can have a higher level of drug in the system compare to other normal people, and a high dose in the blood can lead to drug toxicity.

❒ ADMET-SAR

This website allows you to compute physicochemical descriptors as well as to predict admet parameters, pharmacokinetic properties, drug like nature and medicinal chemistry friendliness of one or multiple small molecules to support drug discovery.

Drug likeness activity were performed and all the compounds obeys Lipinski rule 5 and in the range of drug parameters. Admet analysis shows range of results includes aqueous solubility among the all compounds, Blood brain barrier analysis generally used for penetration studies, level of 0-1 shows high penetration, in this study all the compounds shows high penetration levels hence considered to cross the barrier and act on Central nervous system. CYP450 are the important catalysers for drug metabolism, levels are from 0 and 1.

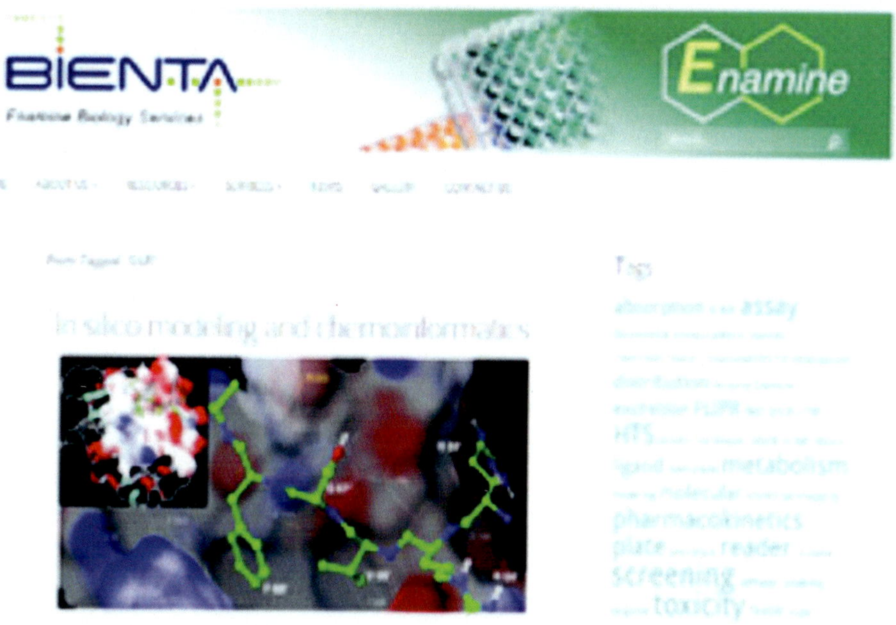

ADME SAR home page

Once the ADMET is over still the scenario need to be very clear because every compound need to qualify some filter which is called as Lipinski rule of five.

Drug likeness activity

A common and simple approach to measure drug-likeness is property-based filters/rules, which define acceptable boundaries of certain molecular physicochemical properties for drugs and/or drug candidates. Finding the drug or the lead is important issue. It is clear that there are different approaches of drug discovery it may mean to generate new chemical structure which has physical and biological properties. Rule of 5 is available by using molsoft software.

In this way a preliminary drug designing process reached to the final step and once the compounds has passed from all the filters the compound can be designate as a DRUG and ready for Clinical trails.

Chapter 9

Genome Analysis in Livestock

D. Chakraborty, Simran Singh, Lopamudra Chakraborty, B. Brahma and D. Kumar

The haploid set of chromosomes in a gamete or microorganism, or in each cell of a mutlicelluar organism is genome. The complete set of genes or genetic material present in a cell or organism is called genome. The genome is the totality of DNA stored in chromosomes typical of each species. The genome contains most of the information needed to specify an organism's properties. The term genome is the combination of gene and chromosome. It represents the entire genetic complement of a prokaryote or virus or the haploid genetic complement of a eukaryote species. With a few minor exceptions, every cell in an animal's body carries the entire genome. Most of the vertebrate genome contains repeated DNA sequences, sequences of unknown function, and sequences which might have no function at all.

Genome analysis approaches

Genome analysis entails the prediction of genes in uncharacterized genomic sequences. The 21st century has seen the announcement of the draft version of the human genome sequence. Model organisms have been sequenced in both the plant and animal kingdoms. A number of different types of technologies have been developed for genome analysis allowing rapid genotyping and genome expression studies using microarray technology. Genome analysis is the identification, measurement or comparison of genomic features such as DNA sequence, structural variation, gene expression or regulatory and functional element annotation at a genomic scale.

Genome analysis has two approaches for identification of genes and characteristics of the genome for understanding and unravelling many of the mysteries for its manipulation in a desired manner. These two main strategies for genome analysis are :

I) Top down

II) Bottom up

Top-down: In the "top-down" approach, a physical map consisting of overlapping large-insert clones (typically BACs) is first constructed and carefully checked. Nowadays, it is often done by STS content mapping, and, in many cases, a proportion of the STSs would have been previously mapped by RH or other methods to provide an additional layer of positional information and to guard against errors in the physical map. In top-down method, a single chromosome is cut (with rare cutter restriction enzymes) into smaller pieces, which are ordered and subdivided; the smaller pieces are then characterized.

Bottom-up: The "bottom-up" approach, conversely, starts with extensive whole-genome shotgun sequencing and assembling of the data into sequence contigs. The bottom up approach involves cutting the chromosome into small pieces, each of which is cloned and ordered. The ordered fragments form contiguous DNA block (contigs). Currently, the resulting "library" of clones varies in sizes from 10, 000 bp to 1Mb. An advantage this approach is the accessibility of these stable clones to other researchers. Contig construction can be verified by FISH, which localizes cosmids to specific regions within chromosomal bands.

1. **Genes: The first markers**

   Since Mendel's time genes have been known or defined in different ways. Such terms as genotype, phenotype, alleles, and different mode of gene interactions elucidate the nature and functions of genes.

2. **DNA Markers**

   The features of genome that are not genes are called DNA markers. Genes are very useful markers but they are by no means ideal as in larger genomes genes are widely spaced out with large gaps between them. There are various approaches to type the DNA sequence features that satisfy this requirement. With the current abundance of massive biological datasets, computational studies have become one of the most important means to biological discovery. Analysis of animal genomes using molecular markers is providing valuable information for breeding programmes to rapidly develop improved livestock breeds with desired productivity. Molecular markers are stable and inherited variations that are measured or detected by a suitable method and are used subsequently to detect the presence of a specific genotype or phenotype other than itself. In conventional genetic analysis there are various types of markers viz. morphological markers, cytogenetic markers, biochemical markers etc. Molecular/DNA marker are the last category to the list of genetical markers. Among all these markers, molecular markers are used extensively in genome analysis studies for the improvement of livestock.

Genome projects typically involve three main phases: DNA sequencing, assembly of DNA to represent original chromosome, and analysis of the representation.

DNA sequencing

DNA sequencing is the process to determine the nucleotide order in a specific DNA molecule, which is useful when attempting to understand its function and consequent effects in the organism it resides in. DNA sequence assembly involves the alignment and merging of DNA fragments to reconstruct the DNA so that smaller sections of the genome can be analyzed. The analysis of DNA phase is the final step in genome analysis. It brings together the discoveries from the previous phases of the project to form conclusions, which can offer true value to further our knowledge of the genome and be applied in relevant situations.

Annotation of DNA

DNA annotation is the process of identifying the locations of genes and coding regions in a genome to create ideas about the possible functions of the genes. There are three main steps to annotate the genome, which include to:

- Identify the portions of the genome that are not involved in coding proteins
- Identify the main elements of the genome (gene prediction)
- Connect the main elements of the genome with biological information

It is important to consider how the genome is similar to other genomes that are already known, as this can help when establishing the role of the gene. Additionally, the plasmids, phages and resistance genes of the genome can reveal information about the nature of the genome. The traditional method of curation method uses the Basic Local Alignment Search Tool (BLAST) algorithm to find similarities to annotate the genome. However, this approach involves expert knowledge and experimental verification to be carried out.

There are also several tools that can automatically annotate the genome *in silico*, which tend to be more efficient than the curation method and can provide additional information. Both curation and technological automation tools are often used together to complement each other in the provision of results.

Technology for genome analysis

Large-scale genome analysis projects are dependent on newly emerging technologies to make the studies practical and economically feasible. For example, the cost of the primers, a significant issue in the past, has been reduced dramatically to make feasible this and other projects that require tens of thousands of oligonucleotides. Other methods of highthroughput analysis are also vital to the success of functional analysis projects, such as microarraying and oligonucleotide chip method.

The recent advances in technology that allow high throughput genomic sequencing to be undertaken quickly and relatively cheaply has propelled the work of genome analysis forward.

However, this progression also places a large demand for efficient and robust tools of analysis to interpret the data into a form that can be utilized in practice. The massive sets of data that have been produced by projects, such as the Human Genome Project, remain largely under-utilized, despite the fact that the project concluded more than a decade ago.

It is important to develop techniques to both analyze the information that we currently have available and the level of data that we are generating. There is currently a lack of robust analysis tools that are able to handle the depth of data in these genome projects and assist researchers in making use of the information.

There are several important functions of the tools used in the process to analyze genomes. The tools should have capabilities to:

- Compare variant calls between genomes
- Export data into convenient formats for analysis
- Filter and annotate results to increase ease of analysis
- Create a reference genome for successive analyses

The development of suitable tools to assist in the genome analysis process should be a priority for the future to continue the growth of knowledge and understanding the field of genomics.

Present status of genome analysis in livestock species

The human genome project has created interest among animal scientists to carryout genome analysis or gene mapping in different animal species. Standing committees have been formulated for various species. Since there is conservation in the genomes particularly in the functional component, the strategies and techniques followed are the same as in humans. A significant progress has been made in many livestock species viz. cattle, buffalo, goat, horse, pigs, poultry etc.

Twenty-three genome sequences are now available in a public database held at the National Center for Biotechnology Information, and numerous genome sequencing projects of a wide variety of organisms, including plants and mammals, are under way.

In animal sciences, DNA markers have been proved as potential and efficient alternate strategy for the problems of identifying and manipulating quantitative trait loci (QTL) in livestock breeding programmes, for study of population genetic structure of phylogeny, pedigree analysis and paternity testing.

Depending upon the nature of molecular information and the particular biological problem addressed, variety of computer software programs are available for analysis.

Genome biotechnology is providing a major opportunity to advance sustainable animal production systems of higher productivity by manipulation of variation within and between breeds. This leads to more rapid and better-targeted gains in breeding value. The molecular markers can enhance the accuracy of selection of sires and can increase the genetic gain 2 to 3 fold.

There is a ample scope that genome analysis in livestock will provide new opportunities to identify genes causative for a number of disorders and will improve our understanding of complex traits for the benefit of livestock and livestock production.

Problems in development of genome analysis in Livestock

Genome analysis in livestock has focused on the molecular identification and characterization of major economical important traits (ETLs=economic trait loci, QTL=quantitative trait loci). As the majority of these traits presumably are regulated by a large number of genes, it is conceivable that up to now QTL mapping has only resulted in the isolation of very few traceable major genes.

There are not many disorders that are of general importance for animal breeding, e.g. stress susceptibility in swine caused by a point mutation in the skeletal muscle ryanodine receptor gene or bovine leukocyte adhesion deficiency caused by a point mutation in the CD18 gene. Therefore, the financial support by breeding organizations or industry is still limited and implementation of DNA-based diagnosis in breeding programs is not only for the improvement of livestock production but also a contribution to animal welfare.

Software Tools for Gene Mapping

Locusmap

Locusmap is a software package designed for rapid linkage analysis and map construction of loci with a variety of inheritance modes. Version 2.1, 08/07/2013. Available for Windows, Linux, and OS X.

GVCeasy

GVCeasy is the graphical user interface for the GVCBLUP package. Version 1.3, 06/20/2014. Available for Windows, Linux, and OS X.

GVCBLUP

GVCBLUP is a software package for genomic prediction and variance component estimation of additive and dominance effects using SNP markers. Version 3.9, 05/12/2014, updated 07/14/2014. Available for Windows, Linux, and OS X.

AGDP

AGDP is a software tool for the analysis of genome differences between populations. Version 1.4, 01/07/2014. Available for Windows and OS X.

SNPEVG	SNPEVG is a graphic tool for SNP effect viewing and graphing of GWAS results. Version 3.2, 11/12/2012. Available for Windows and OS X.
EPISNPmpi	EPISNPmpi is a parallel computing program for epistasis testing in genome-wide association studies for supercomputers and commodity clusters. Version 4.2, 09/16/2011. Available for various parallel computing platforms.
epiSNP	epiSNP is a computer package of serial computing programs for genome-wide testing of SNP epistasis and single-locus effects of complex or quantitative traits. Version 4.2, 09/16/2011, updated 02/06/2012. Available for Windows and Linux.
π_n SPSSQTL	SPSSQTL is a computer program for calculating statistical power and sample size for detecting QTL and candidate gene effects, including single-locus effects and pairwise epistasis effects. Version 1.0, 01/24/2007.
Pedigraph	Pedigraph is a pedigree and genealogy visualization program designed to draw large, complex pedigrees with capability of calculating inbreeding and coancestry coefficients. Version 2.4, 08/19/2008.
MiniInbred	MiniInbred is a program for calculating and minimizing inbreeding coefficients. Version 2.1, 11/17/2014, updated 02/15/2015. Available for Windows, Linux, and OS X.
SHOREmap	Supports genome-wide genotyping and candidate-gene sequencing in a single step through analysis of deep sequencing data from a large pool of recombinants
SIMPLE SImple Mapping PipeLinE	Simplifies the process of mapping new mutations. SIMPLE uses next generation sequencing fastq files to generate tables and plots to show the most likely candidate gene and our locations, with ease
MULTIPOOL	A computational method for genetic mapping in model organism crosses that are analyzed by pooled genotyping.

Mudi Mutation discovery	Detects mutations and prioritizes mutation candidates by analyzing genome re-sequencing data. Mudi also annotates the information of mutations such as gene name and amino acid change.
NGM Next Generation Mapping	Uses a chastity statistic to quantify the relative contribution of the parental mutant and mapping lines to each SNP in the pooled F(2) population.
CloudMap	An accessible and cloud-based pipeline which greatly simplifies the analysis of mutant genome sequences.
SNPTrack	Provides genetic analysis capabilities and captures analysis results in its database as SNP lists that can be cross-linked for biological interpretation to gene/ protein annotations, Gene Ontology

References

Boichard D., Ducrocq V., Fritz S. and Colleau J.J. (2010). Where is Dairy Cattle Breeding Going? A Vision of the Future. Interbull Bulletin No. 41. Paris, France, 63

Colleau, J.J., Fritz, S., Guillaume, F., Baur, A., Dupassieux, D., Boscher, M.Y., Journaux, L., Eggen, A. & Boichard, D. (2009). Simulating the potential of genomic selection in dairy cattle breeding (in French). *Renc Rech Rum, Paris.*

Goddard M E and Hayes B.J. (2007). Genomic Selection. J Anim Breed and Genet. 124: 323-30.

Tantia M S, R K Vijh, V Bhasin, P Sikka, P K Vij, R S Kataria, B P Mishra, S P Yadav, A K Pandey. R K Sethi, B K Joshi, S C Gupta and K M L Pathak. (2011). Whole-genome sequence assembly of the water buffalo (*Bubalus bubalis*). *Indian Journal of Animal Sciences* 81(5): 38–46.

VanRaden, P.M., Van Tassell, C.P., Wiggans, G.R., Sonstegard, T.S., Schnabel, R.D., Taylor, J.F., Schenkel, F.S. (2009). Invited Review: Reliability of Genomic Predictions for North American Holstein Bulls. J. Dairy Sci. **92**: 16-24.

Dekkers, J. C.M. (2012). Application of Genomics Tools to Animal Breeding. *Current Genomics*, **13**: 207-212.

Kutzer, T., Leeb, T. and Brenig, B. (2003). Current State of Development of Genome Analysis in Livestock. 4(6): 487-525. DOI: 10.2174/1389202033490286

https://omictools.com/genetic-mapping-category

https://animalgene.umn.edu/

□□□

Chapter 10

Microsatellites and Analysis of Microsatellite Data

Gyanendra Kumar Rai, Diksha Bhadwal Sreshti Bagati, Vibha Raj Shanti and Rakhshan Jeelani

Microsatellites/SSR/STR

Microsatellites are simple sequence tendem repeats (SSTRs). The repeat units are generally di-, tri-, tetra- or pentanucleotides. For example, a commom rpeat motif in birds is ACn, where the two nucleotides A and C are repeated in bead-like fashion a variable number of times (n could range from 8 to 50). They tend to occur in non-coding regions of DNA (this should be fairly obvious for long dinucleotide repeats) although a few human genetic disorders are caused by flanking regions that consist of "unordered" DNA. The flanking regions are critical because they allow us to develop locus-specific primers to amplify the microsatellites with PCR (polymerase chain reaction). That is, given stretch of unordered DNA 30-50 base pairs (bp) long, the probability of finding that particular stretch more than once in the genome becomes vanishingly small (if the four nucleotides occur with equal probability then the probability of a given stretch 50 bp stretch is 0.2550. In contrast, a given repeat unit (say AC19) may occur in thousands of places in the genome. We use this combination of widely occurring repeat units and locus-specific flanking regions as part of our strategy for finding and developing microsatellite primers. The primers for PCR will be sequences from these unique flanking regions. By having a forward and a reverse primer on each side of the microsatellite, we will be able to amplify a fairly short (100 to 500 bp, where bp means base pair) locus-specific microsatellite region.

Mutation process: microsatellites are useful genetic markers because they tend to be highly polymorphic. It is not uncommon to have human microsatellites with 20 or more alleles and heterozygosities (Hexp = gene diversity, D) of >0.85. Why are they so variable? The reason seems to be that their mutations occur in a fashion very different from that of "classical" point mutations (where a substitution of one nucleotide to another occurs, such as a G substituting for a C). The mutation process in microsatellites occurs through what is known as slippage replication. If we envision the repeat units (e.g., an AC dinucleotide repeat) as beads on a chain, we can imagine that during replication two strands could slip relative positions a bit, but still manage to get zipper going down the beads. One strand or the other could then be lengthened or shortened by addition or excision of nucleotides. The result will be a novel "mutation" that comprises a repeat unit that is one bead longer or shorter than the original. The idea that adding or subtracting one repeat is likely easier than adding or subtracting two or more beads is the basis for using the Stepwise Mutation Model (SMM) as opposed to the Infinite Alleles Model (IAM). An advantage of the SMM (at least in theory) is that the difference in size then conveys additional information about phylogeny of alleles. Under the IAM the only two states are "same" and "different". Under the SMM we have the potential continuum of different similarities (same size, similar in size, very different in size). If, however, the SMM does not hold, then we may be worse off using it- it may actually be highly misleading. Even if the underlying mutation process is largely stepwise, it is not difficult to see how drift might affect the distribution of allele sizes in a way that would almost entirely invalidate the SMM.

Classification of microsatellites

Microsatellites can be classified based on size, the nature of the repeated unit or their position within the genome. With respect to the number of nucleotides per repeat unit, microsatellites can be classified as mono-, di-, tri-, tetra-, penta- or hexa-nucleotide repeats (Table 1). Depending upon the arrangement of nucleotides within the repeat motifs, Weber [1990] used the terms perfect, imperfect and compound to classify microsatellites, whereas Wang *et al.* [2009] coined the terms simple perfect, simple imperfect, compound perfect and compound imperfect. Perfect repeats are tandem arrays of a single repeat motif, whereas imperfect repeats consist of otherwise perfect repeats that are sometimes interrupted by non-repeat sequences. In compound microsatellites, two basic repeat motifs are present together in various configurations. Jarne and Lagoda [1996] coined the terms pure and interrupted to describe perfect or imperfect repeats, respectively, as shown in Table 1.

Table 1. Classification of microsatellites.

A	Based on the arrangement of nucleotides in the repeat motifs	Pure or perfect or simple perfect (CA)*n* Simple imperfect (AAC)*n* ACT (AAC)*n* + 1 Compound or simple compound (CA)*n* (GA)*n* Interrupted or imperfect or compound imperfect (CCA)*n* TT (CGA)*n* + 1
B	Based on the number of nucleotides per repeat	Mononucleotide (A)*n* Dinucleotide (CA)*n* Trinucleotide (CGT)*n* Tetranucleotide (CAGA)*n* Pentanucleotide (AAATT)*n* Hexanucleotide (CTTTAA)*n* (*n* = number of variables)
C	Based on location of SSRs in the genome	Nuclear (nuSSRs) Chloroplastic (cpSSRs) Mitochondrial (mtSSRs)

Comperative Advantages and Disadvantages of Microsatallite Markers

The use of molecular markers is still prohibitively expensive for most large-scale applications in rice breeding programs. Therefore, MAS methods are currently used for more targeted applications [Mackill, 2003]. The advantages and disadvantages of the most commonly used markers are presented in Table 2.

Table 2. Some potential benefits and weakness of the most commonly used markers

S.No.	Markers type	Benefits	Weakness
1.	RFLP	Co-dominant Genomic abundance high Highly reproducible Better genome exposure Applicable across the species No need for sequence information Reliably used in plants	Need high-quality DNA Laborious (compared to RAPD) Complex to automate Radioactive labeling essential Characterization of probe is essential
2.	RAPD	Genomic abundance high Better genome coverage Sequence information unneeded Perfect for automation Requires less DNA No radioactive labeling More rapid	No need of probe information Dominant markers Not reproducible Not suitable for across species Not well tested
3.	SSR	Easy to automate Genomic abundance high Highly reproducible High polymorphism Multiple alleles Moderately genome coverage No radioactive labeling	Not well-examined Cannot suitable across species Sequence information needed
4.	AFLP	High polymorphism Genomic abundance high Can be used across species No need for sequence information Useful in preparing counting maps Works with smaller RFLP fragments	Very tricky due to changes in materials used Not reproducible Very good primers needed
5.	Sequence-tagged site (STS)	Helpful in preparing counting maps Highly reproducible No radioactive labeling Can use filters many times	Need sequence information Out of the target sites, mutation detection not possible Laborious

		Moderate genome coverage	Cloning and probe characterization required
6.	Minisatellites	Highly polymorphic Multiallelic markers High reproducibility Low cost	Many informative bands per reaction Band profiles can not be interpreted in terms of loci and alleles

Source: Kumar et al [2009]

Use of Microsatellites in Agriculture

Microsatellites are useful markers at a wide range of scales of analysis. Until recently, they were most important tool in mapping genomes such as the widely publicized **mapping** of the human genome. They serve a role in biomedical diagnosis as markers for certain disease conditions. That is, certain microsatellite alleles are associated (through genetic linkage) with certain mutations in coding regions of the DNA that can cause a variety of medical disorders. They have also become the primary marker for DNA testing in **forensics** (court) contexts both for human and wildlife cases (e.g., Evett and Weir, 1998). The reason for this prevelance as a forensic marker is their high specificity. Match identities for microsatellite profiles can be very high (probability that the evidence from the crime scene is not a match with that of the suspect is <one in many millions in some cases). In a biological/ evolutionary context they are useful as markers for **parentage analysis.** They can also be used to address questions concerning **degree of relatedness** of individuals or groups. For captive or endangered species, microsatellites can serve as tools to evaluate inbreeding levels (FIS). From there we can move up to the **genetic structure of subpopulations** and populations (using tools such as F-statistics and genetic distances). They can be used to assess **demographic history** (e.g., to look for evidence of population bottlenecks), to assess effective population size (Ne) and to assess the magnitude and directionality of **gene flow between populations**. Microsatellites provide data suitable for **phylogeographic studies** that seek to explain the concordant biogeographic and genetic histories of the flora and faunas of large-scale regions. They are also useful for fine-scale phylogenies up to the level of closely related species. An overview by Selkoe and Toonen (2006) provides a useful practical guide to the use of microsatellites as **geneticmarkers**.

STR plays important role in mapping, trait improvement, variety development, variety identification and product traceability. Traditionally, characterization of varieties is based on phenotypic observation but it is difficult to distinguish varieties with very similar morphological characteristics and identification of the cultivars accurately is essential for maintaining cultivar integrity and Plant Breeders' Rights.

Limited studies have been reported in variety identification of tomato using STR DNA markers. In one study, out of 20 STR markers, only 11 were able to discriminate 47 varieties (Sardaro *et al.,* 2013) and in another study, 12 markers could differentiate 34 varieties (Srivastava *et al.,* 2011). Studies based on 6000 SNP markers over 93 varieties have demonstrated SNP based variety differentiation is also possible (Viquez-Zamora *et al.,* 2013). However, in such SNP based studies, the genotyping data of "Moneymaker" and Moneyberg" varieties were completely identical leading to no differentiation at all. To overcome this Iquebal *et al.,* 2013 has reported more than 1.4 million markers in tomato. DNA fingerprinting is an appropriate tool to track and trace the tomato supply chain, ensuring not only authenticity and integrity of the products but also the absence of any possible genetic contamination by other species or unwanted components (Marmiroli *et al.,* 2003; Marmiroli *et al.,* 2009; Agrimonti *et al.,* 2011).

Such use of STR in plant variety identification is well reported in many crops like barley varieties (Karakousis *et al.,* 2010), S. tuberosum ssp. tuberosum (Kawachuk *et al.,*1990), sugarcane (Manigbas and Villegas, 2004), capsicum (Shirasawa *et al.,* 2013), eggplant (Stagel *et al.,* 2008) and identification of Basmati rice from that of non-Basmati rice (Atchak *et al.,* 2007). Also, the microsatellite STR markers are the method of first choice to complement the DUS (Distinctness, Uniformity and Stability) testing procedure (McCouch *et al.,* 1997; Becher *et al.,* 2000).

Tomato STR database can be a useful tool in MAS programme of tomato improvement (Iquebal *et al.,* 2013). Such use of STR in crop improvement is already reported in sorghum(Wang *et al.,* 2012), tagging stem rust resistance gene Sr35 in wheat (Babiker *et al.,* 2009), *Fusarium* head blight resistance in wheat (Liu and Anderson, 2003), leaf rust resistance gene Lr35 in wheat (Seyfarth *et al.,* 1999) and mapping of resistance gene effective against Karnal bunt pathogen of wheat (Singh *et al.,* 2004). Wheat improvement programs to enhance leaf rust resistance using STR markers has been attempted (Kolmer *et al.*, 2010). STR markers are also used for introgression programs for trait improvement, for example Soltol QTLs in rice. The location of Soltol QTL on chromosomel 1 and identification of additional QTLs associated with salt tolerance is well identified (Thomson *et al.*, 2010).

Limits to utility of microsatellites: Microsatellites DNA is probably rarely useful for higher-level systematics. That is because the mutation rate is too high. Across highly divergent taxa two problems arise. First, the microsatellite primer sites may not be conserved (that is the primers we use for Species A may not even amplify in Species B). Second, the high mutation rate means that homoplasy becomes much more likely—we can no longer safely assume that two alleles identical in state are identical by descent (from a common , meaning shared not abundant, ancestor). As a concrete example imagine two species, each with an AC19 allele that occurs at high frequency. If the populations diverged long ago it becomes increasingly likely that the way those alleles arose took different pathways (e.g., in one species the AC19 arose from an ancestor that went from AC18 to AC19 to AC20 then back to AC19; in the other species the ancestral AC18 went to AC19 and stayed there. Any inferences we make about the species relationships based on the AC19 similarity would be misleading). The identity in state does not correspond to the identity by descent that provides (reliable) phylogenetic signal. A further potential drawback of using microsatellites is that we tend to have relatively few loci to work with (4-20). In some situations, that raises the probability of having a bias due to forces such as selection acting on one or more loci that may give a misleading impression relative to the true pattern of change for the genome as a whole.

Mining of Microsatellites Markers from Genome

Large number of tools are available which are given in the table along with their respective salient features, URL, limitations along with references.

Name,acronym and weblink of the tool	Salient features	Limitations	Refs
Repeatmasker (www.repeat masker.org/)	Available online and stand-alone; mines perfect, imperfect and compound repeats; accepts data in multiple formats; presents statistical analysis; returns flanking sequences; MaskerAid, a performance enhancement is available	Runs only on Unix/Linux systems; not specific for microsatellites	Not published
Sputnik (http://espressosoftware.com/pages/sputnik.jsp and http://cbi.labri.fr/outils/Pise/sputnik.html)	C-language program available online and stand-alone; mines perfect, imperfect and compound repeats; accepts data in multiple formats; improved versions include Modified Sputnik-I and Modified Sputnik-II	Automated statistical analysis files not generated; runs only on Unix/Linux systems; hexanucleotide repeats are not screened	Not published
Tandem Repeat Finder (TRF) (http://tandem.bu.edu/trf/trf.html)	Both online and standalone versions are GUI; mines perfect, imperfect and compound repeats; platform independent	Accepts inputs as fasta files only; automated statistical analysis file not generated (TRAP; www.coccidia.icb.usp.br/trap/[54] can be used); process limitedsize files	Benson (1999)

		only; output files are numerous and difficult to manage	
Repeatfinder (www.cbcb.umd.edu/software/RepeatFinder/)	Available online and stand-alone; mines perfect, imperfect and compound repeats; accepts multiple formats as input	Runs on Unix/Linux systems; not specific for microsatellites	Not published
eQuicktandem (http://bioweb.pasteur.fr/seqanal/interfaces/etandem.html)	Perl script available online and stand-alone; parts of EMBOSS suite; mines perfect, imperfect and compound repeats; accepts input in multiple formats; generates statistics	Runs only on SGI, Irix, Linux, Sun solaris and Tru64 Unix	Not published
REPuter (http://bibiserv.techfak.unibielefeld.de/reputer)	Available online and stand-alone; stand-alone version can handle large genomic sequences; output catalogued in a format similar to BLAST; statistical and graphical analysis provided; excellent connectivity to BLAST, FASTA	Limited capacity of online version; accepts data in fasta/ plain format only; runs only on Unix; not specific for microsatellites	Kurtz *et al.*, (2001)
Simple-Sequence Repeat Identification tool (SSRIT) and Clemson University Genomics Institute Simple-	Perl script available online and stand-alone; platform independent (CUGIssr is a modified version of SSRIT)	Finds only perfect repeats; accepts only fasta-formated files; automated statistical analysis not generated	Temnykh, *et al.*(2001)

Sequence Repeat Tool (CUGIssr) (www.grameneorg/db/searches/ssrtool)			
Tandem Repeats Occurrence Locator (TROLL) (http://wsmartins.net/cgilocal/webtroll/troll.cgi) and WebTROLL (http://wsmartins.net/webtroll/troll.html)	C++program available online and stand-alone (TROLL downloadable, WebTROLL web interface); identifies perfect, imperfect and compound repeats; also designs primers	Accepts fasta-formatted files only as input; executes only on Linux systems; statistical analysis not provided	Castelo, *et al.*(2012)
Microsatellite Analysis Server (MICAS) (http://210.212.212.7/MIC/index.html)	An exclusively web-based utility	Scans only one file at a time; compound and imperfect repeats are not identified; statistical analysis is not performed	Sreenu, *et al.*(2003)
MISA (http://pgrc.ipkgatersleben.de/misa/)	Perl script executing only offline; large sequences are handled easily; statistical analysis is generated; platform independent; can design primers using Primer3 by running supplementary scripts	Inappropriate clustering of microsatellite motifs in statistical analysis file; only fasta-formatted files are taken as input; identifies only perfect repeats and compound repeats	Theil, *et al.* (2003)
mreps (https://bioinfo.lifl.fr/mreps/mreps.php and http://bioweb.pasteur.fr/seqanal/interfaces/mreps.html)	Available online and stand-alone; identifies compound and imperfect repeats; accepts data in multiple formats; platform independent; can design primers	Statistical analysis is not performed	Kolpakov, *et al.*(2003)

Search for Tandem Repeats in Genomes (STRING) (http://www.caspur.it/_castri/STRING/)	C-language program available online and stand-alone; finds perfect, imperfect and compound repeats; runs well with large genomic sequences; platform independent	Only fasta files taken as input; no automated statistical analysis	Parisi, *et al.* (2003)
Search for Tandem Approximate Repeats (STAR) (http://atgc.lirmm.fr/star)	Available online and stand-alone; searches for 'approximate' tandem repeats of a given motif; platform independent	Does not generate statistical analysis	Delgrange and Rivals, (2004)
MicrosatDesign(http://daphnia.cgb.indiana.edu/wfleabase/software)	Perl scripts executing as a stand-alone tool; builds database and design primes from the nascent DNA-sequencer outputs; DNA-seqeunce trace files are taken as an input; combination of phredPhrap, Primer3 and GCG software/e Tandem software; identifies compound repeats and imperfect repeats as well	Specific in its use; does not generate statistical analysis	Singan and Colbourne (2005)
Poly (http://bioinformatics.org/poly/)	Downloadable Python script; statistical analysis is provided; platform independent	Slow	Bizzaro and Marx (2003)

Exact Tandem Repeats Analyzer (E-TRA) and Tandem Repeats Analyzer (TRA) (ftp.akdeniz.edu.tr/Araclar)	C++program available online and stand-alone; search microsatellites in ESTs combining with key-word match searches; multiple sequences and multiple files can be handled simultaneously; provide flanking seque nces and capable of designing primers; fast; GUI; find perfect, imperfect and compound repeats; accept input in multiple formats; provides statistical analysis	Redundancy in output	Karaca (2005)
msatcommander (http://code.google.com/p/msatcommander)	Perl scripts executing online and stand-alone; finds compound repeats and imperfect repeats also; accepts input in multiple formats; statistical analysis can be obtained on executing additional scripts; separate scripts for designing primers	Runs on Unix and Mac OS environment; stand-alone version complicated owing to requirements to execute as many as four scripts for complete analysis	Thursto and Field (2005)
msatcommander (http://code.google.com/p/msatcommander)	Python script available for download; GUI; capable of searching perfect, imperfect and compound repeats with flexibility; output in CSV format;	No online interface; only fasta formatted files accepted as input; statistical analysis is not generated automatically	Fairclot, (2007)

	platform independent; primer designing utility available		
SciRoKo (www.kofler.or.at/bioinformatics/SciRoKo/index.html)	C#-language program available for stand-alone execution; identifies perfect, imperfect and compound repeats, highly flexible; extremely fast; GUI; provides statistical analysis; platform independent	Depends on.NET framework	Kofler, iet al. (2007)
Imperfect Microsatellite Extraction (IMEx) (http://203.197.254.154/IMEX/)	C-language program executing stand-alone; finds perfect and imperfect repeats; efficient, fast and user-friendly; returns the coding/noncoding information of microsatellites; highly flexible; can design primers as well; statistics are generated	Executes on Linux	Mudunuri and Nagarajaram, (2007)

Analysis of microsatallite data

You can also download Word document on Web Genetic software. Luikart and England (1999) provides an (older) overview of approaches. For use of alternative markers see papers (mostly TREE) by Sunnucks (2000), Mueller and Wolfenbarger (1999; AFLP), Campbell *et al.* (2013;AFLP) and Brumfield et al. (2003; SNPs- single nucleotide polymorphisms).

1. Traditional population genetics tools
   - Heterozygosity (Hobs, Hexp = D)
   - Hardy- Weinberg equilibrium
   - Linkage disequilibrium
   - FST and other F- statistics
   - Genetic distances (Cavalli- Sforza chord, Neis 1972 and 1978 distances)
   - Estimates of 4Nem and 4Nem. (m for mutation, m for migration)
2. Microsatellite specific measures (mostly relying on SMM, Stepwise Mutation Models)
   - (delta nu squared) of Goldstein et al. 1995
   - DSW of Shriver *et al.* (1995)
   - RST of Slatkin (1995) as implemented by Goodman (1997)
   - Of Michalakis and Excoffier (1996)
3. Newer phylogeographic and population genetic tools
   - Coalescent inferences (Beerli and Felsenstein, 1999; Rannala and Mountain, 1997)
   - Assignment tests (Davies *et al.*, 1999; software DOH.html)
   - Assessment of whether the population is panmictic or shows distinct partitions (Pritchard *et al.*, 2000 and program structure)
   - Asymmetric migration analyses (Beerli and Felsenstein, 1999)
   - Comparisons and contrasts with maternally inherited mitochondrial DNA structure (Piertney *et al.*, 2000; Chesser and Baker, 1996)
   - Assessment of prior bottlenecks.

References

1. Agrimonti, C., Vietina, M., Pafundo, S., Marmiroli, N. (2011). The use of food genomics to ensure the traceability of olive oil. *Trends Food Sci. Tech,* 22: 237-244.

2. Archak, S., Lakshminarayanareddy, V., Nagaraju, J. (2007). High-throughput multiplex microsatellite marker assay for detection and quantification of adulteration in Basmati rice (*Oryza sativa*). *Electrophoresis,* 28: 2396-2405.

3. Babiker, E., Ibrahim, A.M.H., Yen, Y., Stein, J. (2009). Identification of microsatellite marker associated with stem rust resistance gene *Sr35* in wheat. *Aust J. Crop Sci.,* 3: 195-200.

4. Becher, S.A., Steinmetz, K., Weising, K., Boury, S., Pelteir, D., Renou, J.P., Kahl, g., Wolff, K. (2000). Microsatellites for variety identification in *Pelargonium. Theor. Appl. Genet.,* 101: 643-651.

5. Beerli, P., and Felsenstein, J. (1999). Maximum likelihood estimation of migration rates and population numbers of two populations using a coalescent approach. *Genetics,* 152: 763-773.

6. Benson, G. (1999). Tandem repeats finder: a program to analyze DNA sequences. *Nucleic Acids Res.* 27: 573-580.

7. Bizzaro, J.W. and Marx, K.A. (2003). Poly: quantitative analysis tool for simple sequence repeat (SSR) tracts in DNA. *BMC Bioinformatics,* 4: 22.

8. Blouin, M.S. (2003). DNA-based methods for pedigree reconstruction and kinship analysis in natural populations. *Trends Ecol. Evol.* 18: 503-511.

9. Brumfield, R.T., Beerli, P., Nickerson, D.A. and Edwards, S.V. (2003). The utility of single nucleotide polymorphisms in inferences of population history. *Trends Ecol. Evol.* 18: 249-256.

10. Campbell, D., P. Duchesne, and L. Bernatchez. (2003). AFLP utility for population assignment studies: analytical investigation and empirical comparison with microsatellites. *Mol. Ecol.* 12: 1979-1991.

11. Caastelo, A.T. *et al.* (2002). TROLL - tandem repeat occurrence locator. *Bioinformatics,* 18: 634-636.

12. Chesser, R.K, and R.J. Baker. (1996). Effective sizes and dynamics of uniparentally and diparentally inherited genes. *Genetics,* 144: 1225-1235.

13. Davies, N., F.X. Villablanca, and G.K. Roderick. (1999). Determining the source of individuals: multilocus genotyping in nonequilibrium population genetics. *Trends Ecol. Evol.* 14: 17-21.

14. Delgrange, O. and Rivals, E. (2004). STAR: an algorithm to search for tandem approximate repeats. *Bioinformatics,* 20: 2812-282.

15. Evett, I.W. and B.S. Weir. (1998). Interpreting DNA evidence: Statistical Genetics for Forensic Scientists. Sinauer Associates, Sunderland, MA.

16. Faircloth, B.C. (2007). Msatcommander: detection of microsatellite repeat arrays and automated locus- specific primer design. *s* Notes DOI: 10.1111/j.1471-8286.2007.01884.x (http://blackwellsynergy.com/)

17. Goldstein, D.B., A.R. Linares, L.L. Cavalli-Sforza, and M.W. Feldman. (1995). Genetic absolute dating based on microsatellites and the origin of modern humans. *PNAS USA* 92: 6723-6727.

18. Goodman, S.J. (1997). RST Calc: a collection of computer-programs for calculating estimates of genetic differentiation from microsatellite data and determining their significance. *Mol. Ecol.* 6: 881-885.

19. Hughes, C.R. (1998). Integrating molecular techniques with field methods in studies of social behavior : a revolution results. *Ecology* 79: 383-399.

20. Karaca, M. *et al.* (2005). exact tandem repeats analyzer: A new program for DNA sequence mining. *J. Genet.* 84: 49-54.

21. Karakousis, A., Barr, A.R., Chalmers, K.J., Ablett, G.A., Holton, T.A., Henry, R.J., Lim, P., Langridge, P. (2003). Potential of SSR markers for plant breeding and variety identification in Australian barley germplasm. *Aust. J. of Agri. Res,* 54: 1197-1210.

22. Kawchuk, L.M., Martin, R.F., Mcpherson, J. (1990). Resistance in transgenic potato expressing the potato leafroll virus coat protein gene. *Mol. Plant Microbe In,* 3: 301-307.

23. Kofler, R. *et al.* (2007). SciRoKo: a new tool for whole genome microsatellite search and investigation. *Bioinformatics* 23: 1683-1685.

24. Kolmer, J.A., Anderson, J.A., Flor, J.M. (2010). Chromosome location, linkage with Simple Sequence Repeat Markers, and Leaf Rust Resistance Conditioned by Gene in Wheat. *Crop Sci.,* 50: 2392-2395.

25. Kolpakov, R. *et al.* (2003). Efficient and flexible detection of tendam repeats in DNA. *Nucleic Acids Res.* 31: 3672-3678.

26. Kurtz, S. *et al.* (2001). REPuter: the manifold application of repeats analysis on a genomic scale.*Nucleic Acids Res.* 29: 4633-464.

27. Liu, S., Anderson, J.A. (2003). Marker Assistance Evaluation of *Fusarium* Head Blight Resistance Wheat Germplasm. *Crop Sci.,* 43: 760-766.

28. Manigbas, N.L., Villegas, L.C. (2004). Microsatellite Markers in Hybridity tests to identify true hybrids of sugarcane. *Phillip J. Crop Sci.,* 29(2): 23-32.

29. Marmiroli, N., Maestri, E., Pafundo, S., Vietina, M. (2009). Molecular traceability of olive oil: From plant genomics to food genomics. In Advances in olive resources. Edited by Berti L, Maury J. Trivandrum, India: *Transworld Research Network,* 157-172.

30. Marmiroli, N., Peano, C., Maestri, E. (2003). Advanced PCR techniques in identifying food components. In *Food authenticity and traceability*. Edited by M. Lees. Cambridge UK: *Woodhead Publishing,* 3-33.

31. McCouch, S.R., Chen, X., Panaud, O., Temnykh, S., Xu, Y., Cho, Y.G., Huang, N., Ishii, T., Blair, M. (1997). Microsatellite Marker Development, Mapping and Applications in Rice Genetics and Breeding. *Plant Mol Biol,* 35: 89-99.

32. McDonald, D.B., and W.K. Potts. (1997). Microsatellite DNA as a genetic marker at several scales. pp. 29-49. In Avian Molecular Evolution and Systematics (D. Mindell, ed.). Academics Press New York.

33. Michalakis, Y., and L. Excoffier. (1996). A generic estimation of population subdivision using distances between alleles with special reference for microsatellite loci. *Genetics* 142: 1061-1064.

34. Mudunri, S.B. and Nagarajaram, H.A. (2007). IMEx: Imperfect microsatellite extractor. *Bioinformatics* 23: 1181-1187.

35. Mueller, U.G. and L.L. Wolfenbarger. (1999). AFLP genotyping and fingerprinting. *Trends Ecol. Evol.* 14: 389-394.

36. Parisi, V. *et al.* (2003). STRING: finding tandem repeats in DNA sequences. *Bioinformatics* 19: 1733-1738.

37. Parker, P.G, A.A. Snow, M.D. Schug, G.C. Booton, and P.A. Fuerst. (1998). What molecules can tell us about populations: choosing and using molecular markers.*Ecology* 79: 361-382.

38. Piertney, S.B., A.D.C. MacColl, P.J. Bacon, P.A. Racey, X. Lambin, and J.F. Dallas. (2000). Matrilineal genetic structure and female-

mediated gene flow in red grouse (Lagopus lagopus scoticus): An analysis using mitochondrial DNA. *Evol.* 54: 279-289.

39. Pritchard, J.K., M. Stephens, and P. Donnelly. (2000). Inference of population structure using multilocus genotype data. *Genetics* 155: 945-959.

40. Rannala, Bruce, and J.L. Mountain. (1997). Detecting immigration by using multilocus genotypes. *PNAS* 94: 9197-9201.

41. Sardaro, M.L.S., Marmiroli, M., Maestri, E., Marmiroli, N. (2013). Genetic characterization of Italian tomato varieties and their traceability in tomato food products. *Food Sci. Nutri,* 1(1): 54-62.

42. Selkoe, K.A., and R.J. Toonen. (2006). Microsatellites for ecologists: a practical guide to using and evaluating microsatellite markers. *Ecol. Letters* 9: 615-629.

43. Seyfarth, R., Feuillet, c., Schachermayr, G., Winzeler, M., Keller, B. (1999). Development of a molecular marker for the adult plant leaf rust resistance gene Lr35 in wheat. *Theory Appl. Genet,* 99(3-4): 554-560.

44. Shirasawa, K., Ishii, K., Kim, C., Ban, T., Suzuki, M., Ito, T., Muranaka, T., Kobayashi, M., Nagata, N., Isobe, S., Tabata, S. (2013). Development of Capsicum EST-SSR markers for species identification and in silico mapping onto tomato genome sequence. *Mol. Breeding,* 3(1): 101-110.

45. Shoemaker, J.S. *et al.* (1999). Bayesian statistics in genetics - a guide for the uninitiated. *Trends Genet.* 15: 354-358.

46. Shriver, M.D., L. Jin, E. Boerwinkle, R. Deka, R.E. Ferell, and R. Chakraborty. (1995). A novel measure of genetic distance for highly polymorphic tandem repeat loci. Mol. Boil. Evol. 12: 914-920.

47. Singan, V. and Colbourne, J.K. (2005). MicrostatDesign is a pipeline for transforming sequencer trace files into DNA markers. CGB Technical Report 2005-01. The Centre for Genomics and Bioinformatics, Indiana University, Bloomington. DOI: 10.2506/ cgbtr- 200501.

48. Singh, R., Datta, D., Priyamvada, Singh S, Tiwari, R. (2004). Marker-assisted selection for leaf rust resistance genes *Lr19* and *Lr24* in wheat (*Triticum aestivum* L.). *Appl. Genet,* 45(4): 399-403.

49. Slatkin, M. (1995). A measure of population subdivision based on microsatellite allele frequencies. *Genetics* 139: 457-462.

50. Sreenu, V.B. *et al.* (2003). MICAS: A fully automated web server for microsatellite extraction and analysis from prokaryote and viral genome sequences. *Appl. Bioinformatics* 2: 165-168.

51. Srivastava, D.K., Shoemaker, L.S., Franks, C.E., Sussman, M.D. (2011). Single laboratory validation of a microsatellite marker- based method in tomato variety identification. *J. AOAC Int.* 94(1):251-258.

52. Stagel, A., Portis, E., Toppino, L., Rotino, G.L., Lanteri, S. (2008). Gene- based microsatellite development for mapping and phylogeny studies in eggplant. *BMC Genomics,* 9: 357-370.

53. Strassman, J.E., Solis, C.R., Peters, J.M. and Queller, D.C. (1996). Strategies for finding and using highly polymorphic DNA microsatellite loci for studies of genetic relatedness and pedigrees. Pp. 163-180, In Molecular Zoology: Advances, Strategies and Protocols (J.D. Ferraris, and S.R. Palumbi, eds.). John Willey and Sons, New York. [See also detailed protocols on pp. 558-549].

54. Sunnucks, P. (2000). Efficient genetic markers for population biology. *Trends Ecol. Evol.* 15: 199-203.

55. Temnykh, S. *et al.* (2001). Computational and experimental analysis of microsatellites in rice (*Oryza sativa* L.): Frequency, length variation, transposon associations, and genetic marker potential. *Genome Res.* 11: 1441-1452.

56. Theil, T. *et al.* (2001). Exploiting EST databases for the development of cDNA derived microsatellite markers in barley (*Hordeum vulgare* L.). *Theor. Appl. Genet.* 106: 411-422.

57. Thompson, M.J., de Ocampo, M., Egdane, J., Rahman, M.A., Sajise, A.G., Adorada, D.L., Tumimbang-Raiz, E., Blumwald, E., Seraj, Z.I., Singh, R.K., Gregorio, G.B., Ismail, A.M. (2010). Characterizing the Saltol quantitative trait locus for salinity tolerance in rice. Rice 2010, 3: 148-160.

58. Thurston, M. and Field, D. (2005). Msatminer: detection and characterization of microsatellites. Distributed by the authors at http://www.genomics.ceh.ac.uk/msatfinder/. CEH Oxford, Mansfield Road, Oxford OXI 3SR.

59. Viquez-Zamora, M., Vosman, B., van de Geest, H., Bovy, H., Visser, R.G.F., Finkers, R., van Heusden, A.W. (2013). Tomato breeding in genomics era: insights from a SNP array. *BMC Genomics,* 14: 354.

60. Wang, Y., Bible, P., Loganantharaj, R., Upadhyaya, H.D. (2012). Identification of SSR markers associated with height using pool-

based genome-wide association mapping in sorghum. *Mol. Breeding,* 30(1): 281-292.

61. Weber J.L. (1990). Informativeness of human (dC-dA)*n*(dGdT)*n* polymorphisms. Genomics. 7: 524-530.
62. Wang M.L., Barkley N.A., Jenkins T.M. (2009). Microsatellite markers in plants and insects. Part I. Applications of biotechnology. Genes Genomes Genomics. 3: 54-67.
63. Jarne P., Lagoda P.J.L. (1996). Microsatellites, from molecules to populations and back. Trends Ecol. Evol. 11: 424-429.
64. Kumar P., Gupta V.K., Misra A.K., Modi D.R., Pandey B.K. (2009). Potential of molecular markers in plant biotechnology. Plant Omics J. 2: 141-162.
65. Mackill D.J. (2003). Applications of genomics to rice breeding. IRRN. 28: 9-15.

❑❑❑

Chapter 11

Prediction of Tertiary Protein Structure through Homology Modelling

Budhayash Gautam

The ultimate goal of protein modeling is to predict a structure from its sequence with an accuracy that is comparable to the best results achieved experimentally. This would allow users to safely use rapidly generated in silico protein models in all the contexts where today only experimental structures provide a solid basis: structure-based drug design, analysis of protein function, interactions, antigenic behavior, and rational design of proteins with increased stability or novel functions. In addition, protein modeling is the only way to obtain structural information if experimental techniques fail. Many proteins are simply too large for NMR analysis and cannot be crystallized for X-ray diffraction.

There are three major approaches to three-dimensional (3D) structure prediction for proteins, called as Ab - initio Methods, Comparative or Homology Modelling and Threading Approaches. Among the three major approaches to three-dimensional (3D) structure prediction, homology modeling is the easiest one.

It is based on two major observations

1. The structure of a protein is uniquely determined by its amino acid sequence. Knowing the sequence should, at least in theory, suffice to obtain the structure.
2. During evolution, the structure is more stable and changes much slower than the associated sequence, so that similar sequences adopt practically identical structures, and distantly related sequences still fold into similar structures.

THE SEVEN STEPS TO HOMOLOGY MODELING

In practice, homology modeling is a multistep process that can be summarized in seven steps (Figure 1):

1. Template recognition and initial alignment
2. Alignment correction
3. Backbone generation
4. Loop modeling
5. Side-chain modeling
6. Model optimization
7. Model validation

At almost all the steps choices have to be made. The modeler can never be sure to make the best ones, and thus a large part of the modeling process consists of serious thought about how to gamble between multiple seemingly similar choices.

Step 1: Template Recognition and Initial Alignment

In the safe homology modeling zone, the percentage identity between the sequence of interest and a possible template is high enough to be detected with simple sequence alignment programs such as BLAST or FASTA. To identify these hits, the program compares the query sequence to all the sequences of known structures in the PDB. In practice, one just feeds the query sequence to one of the countless BLAST servers on the web, selects a search of the PDB, and obtains a list of hits-the modeling templates and corresponding alignments.

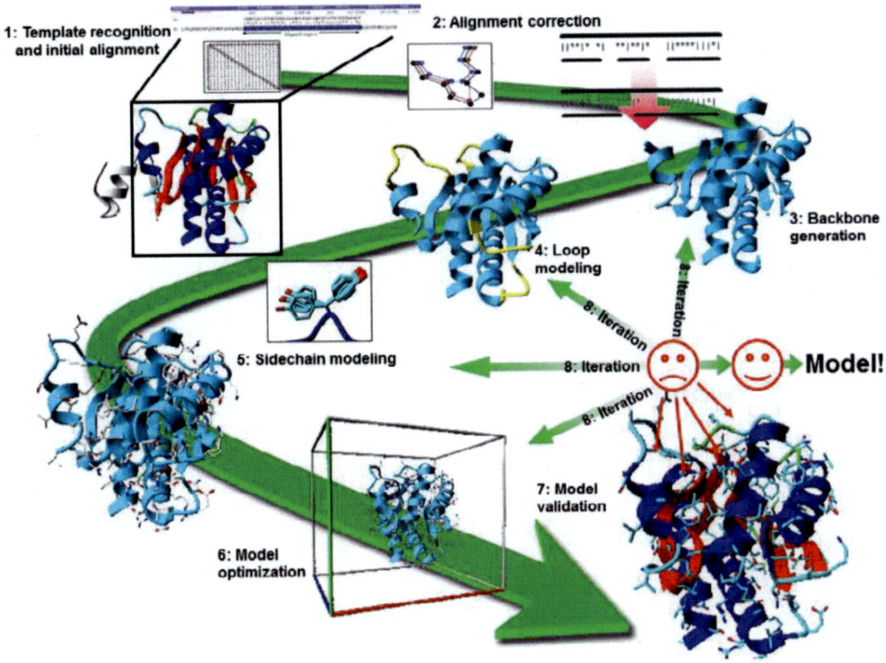

Fig. 1 The steps to homology modeling. The fragment of the template corresponding to the region aligned with the target sequence forms the basis of the model (including conserved side chains). Loops and missing side chains are predicted, then the model is optimized and finally validated.

Step 2: Alignment Correction

Having identified one or more possible modeling templates using the fast methods described above, it is time to consider more sophisticated methods to arrive at a better alignment. Sometimes it may be difficult to align two sequences in a region where the percentage sequence identity is very low. One can then use other sequences from homologous proteins to find a solution.

Step 3: Backbone Generation

When the alignment is ready, the actual model building can start. Creating the backbone is trivial for most of the model: One simply copies the coordinates of those template residues that show up in the alignment with the model sequence. If two aligned residues differ, only the backbone coordinates (N,Cα,C and O) can be copied. If they are the same, one can also include the side chain (at least the more rigid side chains, since rotamers tend to be conserved).

Step 4: Loop Modeling

In the majority of cases, the alignment between model and template sequence contains gaps. Either gaps in the model sequence (deletions) or in the template sequence (insertions). In the first case, one simply omits residues from the template, creating a hole in the model that must be closed. In the second case, one takes the continuous backbone from the template, cuts it, and inserts the missing residues. Both cases imply a conformational change of the backbone. The good news is that conformational changes cannot happen within regular secondary structure elements. It is therefore safe to shift all insertions or deletions in the alignment out of helices and strands, placing them in loops and turns. The bad news is that these changes in loop conformation are notoriously difficult to predict (the big unsolved problem in homology modeling). To make things worse, even without insertions or deletions we often find quite different loop conformations in template and target.

Three main reasons can be identified

1. Surface loops tend to be involved in crystal contacts, leading to a significant conformational change between template and target.
2. The exchange of small to bulky side chains underneath the loop pushes it aside.
3. The mutation of a loop residue to proline or from glycine to any other residue. In both cases, the new residue must fit into a more restricted area in the Ramachandran plot, which most of the time requires conformational changes of the loop.

There are two main approaches to loop modeling

1. Knowledge based: one searches the PDB for known loops with endpoints that match the residues between which the loop has to be inserted, and simply copies the loop conformation. All major molecular modeling programs and servers support this approach (e.g., 3D-Jigsaw, Insight, Modeller, Swiss-Model, or WHAT IF).
2. Energy based: as in true ab initio fold prediction, an energy function is used to judge the quality of a loop. Then this function

is minimized, using Monte Carlo or molecular dynamics techniques to arrive at the best loop conformation. Often the energy function is modified (e.g., smoothed) to facilitate the search.

Step 5: Side-Chain Modeling

When we compare the side-chain conformations (rotamers) of residues that are conserved in structurally similar proteins, we find that they often have similar ÷ 1 -angles (i.e., the torsion angle about the C α"C β bond). It is therefore possible to simply copy conserved residues entirely from the template to the model (see also Step 3) and achieve a higher accuracy than by copying just the backbone and repredicting the side chains.

Step 6: Model Optimization

The problem just mentioned above leads to a classical chicken-and-egg situation. To predict the side-chain rotamers with high accuracy, we need the correct backbone, which in turn depends on the rotamers and their packing. The common approach to such a problem is an iterative one: predict the rotamers, then the resulting shifts in the backbone, then the rotamers for the new backbone, and so on, until the procedure converges.

The most straightforward approach to model optimization is simply to run a molecular dynamics simulation of the model. Such a simulation follows the motions of the protein on a femtosecond (10 "15 s) timescale and mimics the true folding process. One thus hopes that the model will complete its folding and "home in" to the true structure during the simulation. The advantage is that a molecular dynamics simulation implicitly contains entropic effects that are otherwise difficult to treat; the disadvantage is that the force fields are again not precise enough to make it work.

Step 7: Model Validation

Every homology model contains errors. The number of errors (for a given method) mainly depends on two values:

1. The percentage sequence identity between template and target. If it is greater than 90%, the accuracy of the model can be compared to crystallographically determined structures, except

for a few individual side chains (Chothia and Lesk, 1986; Sippl, 1993). From 50% to 90% identity, the rms error in the modeled coordinates can be as large as 1.5 Å, with considerably larger local errors. If the sequence identity drops to 25%, the alignment turns out to be the main bottleneck for homology modeling, often leading to very large errors.

2. The number of errors in the template.

   Errors in a model become less of a problem if they can be localized. It is, for example, hardly important that a loop far away from an enzyme's active site is placed incorrectly. An essential step in the homology modeling process is therefore the verification of the model.

There are two principally different ways to estimate errors in a structure

1. Calculating the model's energy based on a force field: This method checks if the bond lengths and bond angles are within normal ranges, and if there are lots of bumps in the model (corresponding to a high Van der Waals energy). Essential questions such as "Is the model folded correctly"?

2. Determination of normality indices that describe how well a given characteristic of the model resembles the same characteristic in real structures. Many features of protein structures are well suited for normality analysis. Most of them are directly or indirectly based on the analysis of interatomic distances and contacts.

Summary

In summary, it is safe to say that homology modeling is unfortunately not as easy as stated in the beginning. Ideally, homology modeling uses threading to improve the alignment, and ab initio folding to predict the loops and molecular dynamics simulations with a perfect force field to home in to the true structure.

Protein Modeling Resources

SWISS-MODEL	http://swissmodel.expasy.org
Modeller	http://www.salilab.org
WhatIf	http://www.cmbi.kun.nl/whatif/

3D-JIGSAW	http://www.bmm.icnet.uk/people/paulb/3dj/form.html
CPHmodels	http://www.cbs.dtu.dk/services/CPHmodels/
SDSC1	http://cl.sdsc.edu/hm.html
Some useful Evaluation Tools	
ANOLEA	http://protein.bio.puc.cl/cardex/servers/anolea/
	http://swissmodel.expasy.org/anolea/
ProCheck	http://www.biochem.ucl.ac.uk/~roman/procheck/procheck.html
WhatCheck	http://www.cmbi.kun.nl/gv/whatcheck/
Verify3D	http://www.doe-mbi.ucla.edu/Services/Verify_3D/
Biotech Validation Suite for Protein Structures	http://biotech.ebi.ac.uk:8400/

Reference

Mainly Adapted from "Structural Bioinformatics" Edited by Philip E. Bourne and Helge Weissig ISBN 0-471-20199-5 Copyright @ 2003 by Wiley-Liss, Inc.

About the Authors

Dr. Biswajit Brahma is M.V.Sc. Gold Medallist from National Dairy Research Institute, Deemed University, Karnal, India. He received Ph.D. in Animal Biotechnology from National Dairy Research Institute, and is currently serving as Assistant Professor (SS) in Sher-e-Kashmir University of Agricultural Sciences and Technology of Jammu. Working in the field of animal genomics, Dr. Brahma's research interests include genomic basis of pathogen-host interactions to explain disease resistance in animals, molecular recognition of microbial signatures by pattern recognition receptors and downstream signalling processes for development of non-infectious synthetic vaccine targeting innate immune system and comparative genomics of innate immune receptors and elucidation of mechanism of MAMP recognition by PRR receptors. Author of more than 20 international journal articles, Dr. Brahma has made significant contribution in research through exploration of genetic diversity of innate immune genes of Indian livestock, DNA based methods for detection of cross-species adulteration in animal products, and genetic basis of fecundity and male infertility in Indian livestock.

Dr. Dhirendra Kumar is Ph.D., and is currently serving as Assistant Professor (SS) in Sher-e-Kashmir University of Agricultural Sciences and Technology of Jammu. He has experience of teaching of undergraduate and postgraduate biostatistics courses for over eight years. Dr.Dhirendra has authored more than 30 scientific research papers in reputed national and international journals and six book chapters. He is ex-founder Associate Editor of International Journal of Bioinformatics and Biological Sciences. Dr.Dhirendra, for his professional contribution, has been honoured with Young Scientist Award twice, Distinguished Scientist Award and Excellence in Teaching Award by recognized professional societies.